Never Forget

MICHEL BUSSI

Translated from French by Shaun Whiteside

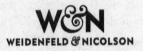
WEIDENFELD & NICOLSON

First published in Great Britain in 2020 by Weidenfeld & Nicolson
This paperback edition published in 2021 by Weidenfeld & Nicolson
an imprint of The Orion Publishing Group Ltd
Carmelite House, 50 Victoria Embankment
London EC4Y 0DZ

An Hachette UK Company

First published in France as *N'oublier jamais* by Presses de la Cité 2014

1 3 5 7 9 10 8 6 4 2

A CIP catalogue record for this book is
available from the British Library.

ISBN (Paperback) 978 1 4746 0184 9
ISBN (eBook) 978 1 4746 0185 6

Typeset by Input Data Services Ltd, Somerset

Printed in Great Britain by Clays Ltd, Elcograf S.p.A.

www.weidenfeldandnicolson.co.uk
www.orionbooks.co.uk

To Arthur . . . 18 tomorrow!

You come across a pretty girl on a cliff edge,
Don't reach out to her!
People might think you've pushed her.

Fécamp, 13 July 2014

From: Lieutenant Bertrand Donnadieu, National Gendarmerie, Territorial Brigade of the District of Étretat, Seine-Maritime

To: M. Gérard Calmette, Director of the Disaster Victim Identification Unit (DVIU), Criminal Research Institute of the National Gendarmerie, Rosny-sous-Bois

Dear Monsieur Calmette,

At 2.45 a.m. on 12 July 2014, a section of cliff of about 45,000 cubic metres collapsed above Valleuse d'Etigues, 3 km west of Yport. Rockfalls of this type are not uncommon on our coast. The emergency services arrived on the scene an hour later and established beyond a doubt that there no casualties resulting from this incident.

However, and this is the reason for this letter, while no walkers were caught in the landslide, the first responders made a strange discovery. Lying among the debris scattered over the beach were three human skeletons.

Police officers dispatched to the site found no personal effects or items of clothing in the vicinity that would enable them to identify the victims. It's possible that they might have been cavers who became trapped; the network of karst caves beneath the famous white cliffs are a popular attraction. However no cavers have been reported missing in recent months, or indeed years. We have analysed the bones with the limited equipment at our disposal and they do not appear to be very old.

I should add that the bones were scattered over forty metres of beach as a result of the landslide. The Departmental Brigade of Forensic Investigation, under the auspices of Colonel Bredin, pieced together the skeletons. Their initial analysis confirms our own: not all of the bones seem to have reached the same level of decomposition. Bizarre as it may seem, this suggests the three individuals had died in that cavity in the cliff at different times, probably several years apart. The cause of their death remains unknown: during our examination of the remains we found no trauma that would have proved fatal.

With no evidence to go on, ante or post mortem, we are unable to pursue the usual lines of inquiry that would allow us to determine who these three individuals were. When they died. What killed them.

The local community, recently unnerved by a macabre event that has no apparent connection to the discovery of these three unidentified corpses, is understandably rife with speculation.

Which is why, Director, while I am aware of the number of urgent matters requiring your attention, and the suffering of those awaiting formal identification of deceased relatives, I would ask you to make this case a priority so that we may proceed with our investigation.

Yours sincerely,

Lieutenant Bertrand Donnadieu,

Territorial Brigade of the District of Étretat

Five months earlier

19 February 2014

'Watch out, Jamal, the grass will be slippery on the cliff.'

André Jozwiak, landlord of the Hotel-Restaurant Sirène, issued the caution before he could stop himself. He'd put on a raincoat and was standing outside his front door. The mercury in the thermometer that hung above the menu was struggling to rise above the blue line indicating zero. There was hardly any wind, and the weathervane – a cast-iron sailing ship fixed to one of the beams on the façade –seemed to have frozen during the night.

The drowsy sun dragged itself wearily above the sea, illuminating a light coating of frost on the cars parked outside the casino. On the beach in front of the hotel the pebbles huddled together like shivering eggs abandoned by a bird of prey. Beyond the final towering sea stack lay the coast of Picardy, a hundred kilometres due east.

Jamal passed the front of the casino and, taking brisk, short strides, set off up Rue Jean-Hélie. André watched him go, blowing on his hands to warm them up. It was almost time to serve breakfast to the few customers who spent their winter holidays overlooking the Channel. At first the landlord had thought the young disabled Arab was odd, running along the footpath every morning, with one muscular leg and one that ended in a carbon foot wedged into a trainer. Now, he felt genuine affection for the boy. When he was still in his twenties, Jamal's age, André used to cycle over a hundred kilometres every Sunday morning, Yport–Yvetot–Yport, three hours with no one pestering him. If this kid from Paris with

3

his weird foot wanted to work up a sweat at first light – well, he understood.

Jamal's shadow reappeared briefly at the corner of the steps that rose towards the cliffs, before disappearing behind the casino wheelie bins. The landlord took a step forward and lit a Winston. He wasn't the only one braving the cold: in the distance, two silhouettes stood out against the wet sand. An old lady holding an extending lead with a ridiculous little dog – the kind that looks as if it runs on batteries, operated by remote control, and so conceited that it goaded the seagulls with hysterical yaps. Two hundred metres further on, a tall man, hands in the pockets of a worn brown leather jacket, stood by the sea, glowering at the waves as if he wanted to take revenge on the horizon.

André spat out the butt of his cigarette and went back into the hotel. He didn't like to be seen unshaven, badly dressed, his hair a mess, looking like the sort of caveman Mrs Cro-Magnon would have walked out on many moons ago.

His steps keeping to a metronomic rhythm, Jamal Salaoui was climbing one of the highest cliffs in Europe. One hundred and twenty metres. Once he'd left the last of the houses behind, the road dwindled to a footpath. The panorama opened up to Étretat, ten kilometres away. Jamal saw the two silhouettes at the end of the beach, the old woman with the little dog and the man staring out to sea. Three gulls, perhaps frightened by the dog's piercing cries, rose from the cliff and blocked his path before soaring ten metres above him.

The first thing Jamal saw, just past the sign pointing to the Rivage campsite, was the red scarf. It was fixed to the fence like a danger sign. That was Jamal's first thought:

Danger.

A warning of a rockfall, a flood, a dead animal.

The idea passed as swiftly as it had come. It was just a scarf caught on barbed wire, lost by a walker and carried away by the wind coming off the sea.

4

Reluctant to break the rhythm of his run, to pause for a closer look at the dangling fabric, he almost carried straight on. Everything would have turned out quite differently if he had.

But Jamal slowed his pace, then stopped.

The scarf looked new. It gleamed bright red. Jamal touched it, studied the label.

Cashmere. Burberry . . . This scrap of fabric was worth a small fortune! Jamal delicately detached the scarf from the fence and decided that he would take it back to the Sirène with him. André Jozwiak knew everyone in Yport, he would know if someone had lost it. And if it wasn't claimed, Jamal would keep it. He stroked the fabric as he continued his run. Once he was back home in La Courneuve, he doubted he would risk wearing it over his tracksuit. In his neighbourhood, someone would rip your head off for a €500 cashmere scarf! But he would no doubt find a pretty girl who'd be happy to wear it.

As he drew near the blockhouse, to his right a small flock of sheep turned their heads in his direction. They were waiting for the grass to thaw with a lobotomised look which reminded him of the idiots that he worked with, standing by the microwave at lunchtime.

Just past the blockhouse, Jamal saw the girl.

He immediately gauged the distance between her and the edge of the cliff. Less than a metre! She was standing on the precipice, looking down at a sheer drop of over a hundred metres. His brain reeled, calculating the risks: the incline to the void, the frost on the grass. The girl was more at risk here than she would have been standing on the ledge of the highest window of a thirty-storey building.

'Mademoiselle, are you all right?'

Jamal's words were snatched away by the wind. No response.

He was still a hundred and fifty metres from the girl.

Despite the intense cold, she was wearing only a loose red dress torn into two strips, one floating over her navel and then to her thighs, the other yawning from the top of her neck to the base of her chest, revealing the fuchsia cup of a bra.

She was shivering.

5

Beautiful. Yet for Jamal there was nothing erotic about this image. Surprising, moving, unsettling, but nothing sexual. When he thought about it later, trying to fathom it out, the nearest equivalent that came to mind was a vandalised work of art. A sacrilege, an inexcusable contempt for beauty.

'Are you all right, mademoiselle?' he said again.

She turned towards him. He stepped forward.

The grass came halfway up his legs, and it occurred to him that the girl mightn't have noticed the prosthesis fixed to his left leg. He was now facing her. Ten metres between them. The girl had moved closer to the precipice, standing with her back to the drop.

He could see that she'd been crying; her mascara had run, then dried. Jamal struggled to marshal his thoughts.

Danger.

Emergency.

Above all, emotion. He felt overwhelmed by emotion. He had never seen such a beautiful woman. Her features would be imprinted on his memory for ever: the perfect oval of her face, framed by twin cascades of jet-black hair, her coal-black eyes and snow-white skin, her eyebrows and mouth forming thin, sharp lines, as if traced by a finger dipped in blood and soot. He wondered whether he was in shock, whether this was impacting on his assessment of the situation, the distress of this stranger, the need to grab her hand without waiting for an answer.

'Mademoiselle . . .'

He held out his hand.

'Don't come any closer,' the girl said.

It was more a plea than an order. The embers in her coal-black irises seemed to have been extinguished.

'OK,' Jamal stammered. 'OK. Stay right where you are, let's take this nice and slow.'

Jamal's eye slipped over her skimpy dress. She must have come out of the casino a hundred metres below. Of an evening, the hall of the Sea View turned into a discotheque.

A night's clubbing that had gone wrong? Tall, slim and sexy, she would have drawn plenty of admirers. Clubs were full of creeps who came to check out the babes.

Jamal spoke as calmly as he could:

'I'm going to step forward slowly, I want you to take my hand.'

The young woman lowered her gaze for the first time and paused at the sight of the carbon prosthesis. This drew an involuntary look of surprise, but she regained control almost immediately.

'If you take so much as a step, I'll jump.'

'OK, OK, I won't move . . .'

Jamal froze, not even daring to breathe. Only his eyes moved, from the girl who had emerged from nowhere, to the orange dawn on the edge of the horizon.

A bunch of drunks following her every move on the dance floor, Jamal thought. And among them, at least one sick bastard, maybe several, perverted enough to follow the girl when she left. Hunt her down. Rape her.

'Has . . . has someone hurt you?'

She burst into tears.

'You could never understand. Keep running. Go! Get out of here, now!'

An idea . . .

Jamal put his hands around his neck. Slowly. But not slowly enough. The girl recoiled, took a step backwards, closer to the drop.

Jamal froze. He wanted to catch her in his hand as if she were a frightened sparrow that had fallen from the nest, unable to fly.

'I'm not going to move. I'm just going to throw you my scarf. I'll hold one end. You grab the other, simple as that. It's up to you whether to let go or not.'

The girl hesitated, surprised once again. Jamal took the opportunity to throw one end of the red cashmere scarf. Two metres separated him from the suicidal young woman.

The fabric fell at his feet.

She leaned forward delicately and, with absurd modesty pulled at the remains of her dress to cover her bare breast, then stood, clutching the end of Jamal's scarf.

'Easy does it,' Jamal said. 'I'm going to pull on the scarf, wrap it

7

around my hands. Let yourself be dragged towards me, two metres, just two metres further from the edge.'

The girl gripped the fabric more tightly.

Jamal knew then that he had won, that he had done the right thing, throwing this scarf the way a sailor throws a lifebelt to someone who's drowning, drawing them gently to the surface, centimetre by centimetre, taking infinite care not to break the thread.

'Easy does it,' he said again. 'Come towards me.'

For a brief moment he realised that he had just met the most beautiful girl he had ever seen. And that he had saved her life.

That was enough to make him lose concentration for one tiny second.

Suddenly the girl pulled on the scarf. It was the last thing Jamal had expected. One sharp, swift movement.

The scarf slid from his hands.

What followed took less than a second.

The girl's gaze fixed on him, indelibly, as if she were looking at him from the window of a passing train. There was a finality to that gaze.

'Noooo!' Jamal shouted.

The last thing he saw was the red cashmere scarf floating between the girl's fingers. A moment later she toppled into the void.

So did Jamal's life, but he didn't know it yet.

I
Instruction

I

Instruction

1

Jamal Salaoui's diary

For a long time, I was unlucky.

Fortune never favoured me. I came to imagine life as a huge conspiracy, with the whole world against me. And at the heart of this conspiracy was a god who behaved like a sadistic teacher, preying on the weakest kid in the class. Meanwhile the rest of the class, only too happy not to be on the receiving end, joined in. From a distance, to avoid getting caught in the crossfire. As if bad luck was contagious.

Then, over the years, I came to understand.

It's an illusion.

In life, the most vicious god you're likely to meet is a teacher who treats you as a scapegoat.

Gods, like teachers, don't give a damn about you. You don't exist for them.

You're on your own.

If you want things to go your way, you have to keep playing the game. You have to pick yourself up and start over, again and again.

Keep trying.

It's the law of probability. And perhaps, at the end of the day, of luck.

My name is Jamal.

Jamal Salaoui.

Not the kind of name that brings good luck, apparently.

Although . . .

My first name, you may have noticed, is the same as that of Jamal Malik, the boy in *Slumdog Millionaire*. And that's not the only thing we have in common. We are both Muslims in a country that is not, and we don't give a toss. He grew up in Dharavi, a Bombay slum, and I grew up in the Barre Balzac – the 'Cité des 4000' – in La Courneuve. I don't know if you can really compare the two of us. Even physically. He isn't very handsome, with his sticky-out ears and his scared-sparrow expression. Neither am I. Worse, I've only got one leg, or rather one and a half; the second ends at the knee with a flesh-coloured plastic-and-carbon prosthesis. I'll tell you about it one day.

It was one of those times when luck wasn't on my side.

But the main point we have in common is standing right in front of me. Jamal Malik's greatest prize isn't the millions of rupees, it's Latika, his sweetheart, pretty as a picture, particularly at the end, with her yellow veil, when he finds her again at Bombay station. She's his jackpot.

I'm the same.

The incredibly desirable girl sitting across from me has just put on a blue tulip dress. Her breasts dance under the silk of a low-cut neckline that I'm allowed to plunge my eyes into for as long as I like. How can I put it so you'll understand? She's my feminine ideal. It's as if she had been flirting with me in my dreams night after night before appearing in front of me one fine morning.

I'm having dinner with her.

At her place.

The glow of the fire in the hearth caresses her pale skin. We're drinking champagne: Piper-Heidsieck 2005. We will make love in a few hours, or perhaps even before the end of the meal.

We will be lovers for at least one night.

Perhaps several.

Perhaps every night for the rest of my life, like a dream that doesn't evaporate in the morning but accompanies me into the shower, then in the lift in the last block in the Cité des 4000 that hasn't been blown up, then all the way to Courneuve-Aubervilliers station where I'll board the RER B line.

She smiles at me. She lifts the champagne glass to her lips, I imagine the bubbles going down into her body, sparkling inside her. I rest my lips on hers. Moist with Piper-Heidsieck like a fizzy sweet.

She chose the intimacy of her home over the elegance of a restaurant by the sea. Perhaps in the end she was a bit ashamed to be seen out with me, wary of the people at the next table seeing a disabled Arab out with the most beautiful girl in the whole region. I understand, even if I don't give a damn about their petty jealousy. I deserve this moment more than anyone. I've staked everything on it. All those times luck didn't go my way, I kept playing the game. And I never stopped believing.

I've won.

I first met this girl six days ago, in the most unlikely place to meet a fairy: Yport.

During those six days, I almost died several times.

I'm alive.

During those six days I was accused of murder. Of several murders. The most sordid crimes you can imagine. I almost believed it myself.

I'm innocent.

I've been hunted down. Judged. Sentenced.

I'm free.

You will see, you too will find it hard to believe the ramblings of a poor disabled Arab. The miracle will seem too unlikely. The cops' version will seem much more plausible. You'll see, you too will doubt me. Right to the end.

You'll come back to the start of this story, you'll reread these lines and you'll think I'm mad, that I'm setting a trap for you, or that I've made it all up.

But I haven't made anything up. I'm not mad. No trap. I'm just asking one thing of you: that you trust me. To the end.

It'll all turn out fine, you'll see.

It's 24 February 2014. It all started ten days ago, one Friday evening, 14 February, just as the kids from the Saint Antoine Therapeutic Institute were leaving for home.

2

Trust me to the end?

Out of nowhere, rain began to fall on the three red-brick buildings of the Saint Antoine Therapeutic Institute of Bagnolet, on the three-hectare park and on the white statues of generous, illustrious and forgotten donors of centuries gone by. A dozen silhouettes stirred abruptly, giving the illusion that the shower was bringing the sculptures to life. Doctors, nurses and stretcher-bearers in white coats ran for shelter like ghosts worried about getting their shrouds wet.

Some took refuge under the porch, others in the twenty or so cars, minivans and minibuses parked one behind the other on the gravel avenue, their doors still open, kids crammed inside.

As always on a Friday evening, the less severely disabled teenagers were heading off to spend the weekend with their families. This particular Friday they could look forward to a weekend plus two weeks holiday.

As soon as I'd deposited Grégory in the back seat of the Scenic, I abandoned his empty wheelchair in the downpour and joined the others in running for shelter. Three cars away, its revolving lights sweeping the rain, was the ambulance; I peered through the rain, trying to see Ophélie, then headed back to the carers' area.

It was like entering one of those picnic rooms for skiers in the mountains. The predominantly female staff of the Saint Antoine Institute – nurses, teachers and psychotherapists – were sitting with their frozen fingers wrapped around mugs of tea or coffee.

Some flicked a glance in my direction, others ignored me; Sarah and Fanny, the youngest teachers, smiled at me, Nicole, the chief shrink, let her gaze linger on my artificial leg, as always. Most of the girls at the Institute liked me, to varying degrees depending on their age, whether they were in a relationship, and their professional conscience. The Mother Teresas outnumbered the Marilyns.

That arsehole Jérôme Pinelli, the section head, came in after me. He scanned the room, and then looked me up and down like a cop.

'They're loading Ophélie in the ambulance. Are you proud of yourself?'

Not really.

I pictured the blue revolving light in the courtyard. Ophélie howling at them to leave her alone. I tried without success to come up with a few words of explanation, or at least of apology. Then I looked around the room for help, knowing I wouldn't find any. My colleagues lowered their heads.

'We'll sort it out after the holidays,' Pinelli concluded.

To the list of everyday torturers in search of a victim, to the vicious gods and sadistic teachers, we must add little fascist bosses like Jérôme Pinelli. Fifty-three. HR manager. Less than six months in the job and already he was responsible for one case of adultery, two depressions and three dismissals.

He went and stood in front of the big poster of Mont Blanc that I'd hung on the wall of the staff room. One metre by two. The entire massif: Mont Blanc, Mont Maudit, Aiguille du Midi, Dent du Géant, Aiguille Verte . . .

'Damn,' Pinelli said, 'it's good to be rid of those stupid teenagers. Oh well, in less than ten hours I'll be in Courchevel . . .'

He turned slowly on his heel as if to let the ladies admire his profile, then came and stood in front of me and stared pointedly at my prosthesis.

'What about you? Off to the snow, Salaoui? Cool. With your carbon foot you only need to hire one ski!'

He burst out laughing, but he was on thin ice; his audience of female carers were hesitant about joining in. The Marilyns chuckled,

15

the Mother Teresas were silently outraged.

Before he could dig himself in any deeper, the opening bars of 'I Gotta Feeling' rang out from his pocket. He took out his phone, grunted 'Fuck!', then sauntered out, addressing me over his shoulder:

'When you get back we'll have to sort this one out, Salaoui. She's a minor, I can't always cover for you.'

Arsehole!

At that moment, Ibou came in and shut the door in his face.

Ibou was my only real ally. A stretcher-bearer at the Institute, it was also his job to put the inmates in straitjackets or get between them when they lost control. Sometimes he helped me with chores like setting up scaffolding, moving furniture around, or changing the tyre on a wheelchair. Ibou was built like a tank carved from a baobab tree. Think Omar Sy. Both the Marilyns and the Mother Teresas were in agreement: that bastard was handsome, cool and funny. Athletic, too.

They weren't aware that when the two of us ran the fifteen kilometres from the Parc de la Courveuve to the Forêt de Montmorency every Thursday, I always finished half a lap ahead of him in the final sprint.

He gave me a high five.

'I heard that jerk and his dig about skiing. Joking aside, Jam, are you going on holiday?'

He turned towards the Mont Blanc poster, looking at it with yearning.

'I'm heading to Yport.'

'Yport? Whoa! Are there any slopes?'

'It's a village in Normandy, big man. Near Étretat. A thousand-metre climb over ten kilometres. But no snow or ski lifts . . .'

Ibou whistled, then addressed the female carers:

'Don't be fooled by appearances, my man Jamal here is a top athlete! This mule of a guy could be a contender in the Paralympics, claiming glory and medals for the Saint Antoine Institute, but he's got it into his head that he wants to be the first one-legged athlete to run the Mont Blanc Ultra-Trail . . .'

I immediately felt a shift in the way the women looked at me. Ibou went on:

'The hardest race in the world. There's no stopping this one, is there?'

The women's eyes darted between me and the poster. In my mind's eye, I was riding the Aiguille du Midi cable car, three thousand metres above sea level, looking down on Mer de Glace . . . Vallorcine. The UTMB – the Ultra-Trail Mont Blanc – was a sixty-eight kilometre run, with an elevation gain of around 9,600 metres, taking around forty-six hours . . . On one leg. Was I capable of such a feat? Pushing myself to the limit, until I forgot my pain? Tears were glistening in the carers' eyes; they were already feeling sorry for me. I felt myself blushing like a virgin. I turned my gaze to the wall, focusing intently on the dirty white plaster, the traces of mould and rust from the leaking ceiling.

'And Jam's a single guy,' Ibou went on. 'Doesn't one of you want to go with him? Forget that Yport crap!'

He winked in my direction. I was standing by.

'Come on, girls,' he urged. 'One volunteer! A week of your dreams, keeping company with an Olympic champion, hitting those glorious heights with him.'

Thanks to Ibou, I felt unstoppable. Then he added:

'Only joking, ladies. You've got to hand it to me, I got you this time!'

3

Until I forget my pain?

Lying at my feet, the corpse slept on a bed of pebbles.

The blood flowed gently under her head, forming a red silk sheet pulled by an invisible hand, a scarlet wave that flowed softly towards the sea.

Even in death, the stranger was incredibly beautiful. Her jet-black hair covered her cold, white face like seaweed clinging to a rock polished by successive tides. The girl's body had become one more fallen piece of cliff that the sea would sculpt until it melted into the décor, for eternity.

My gaze shifted from the body to the towering chalk cliff. In the three days I'd spent in Yport, those cliffs had never seemed so high. Streams of clay from the meadows above left trails on the rockface, like the stains left by rust, damp and dirt on a prison wall. This was a wall put there by the gods to keep mortals from escaping; to jump the wall would mean losing one's life.

I checked my watch: 8.28.

Less than a quarter of an hour had passed since I had left the Sirène for my daily run. I thought again of the landlord's advice:

Watch out, Jamal, the grass will be slippery on the cliff.

And then the red scarf caught on the fence, the sheep, the block-house . . . the pictures flowed together, one after another. I saw the girl on the edge of the precipice, her torn dress, her last words, 'Don't come any closer . . . You could never understand.' The unfathomable desolation on her face before she toppled into the void, the Burberry cashmere scarf that I had held out to her, clutched in her fist.

My heart went on thumping in time with my frantic race, right after she jumped, all the way to the beach, as if I could have got there before her, caught her in my arms.

Ridiculous.

'I saw her fall,' murmured a sombre voice behind me.

It was the man in the brown leather jacket. He approached the body with obvious reluctance.

'I heard you yell,' he said in the same weary voice. 'I turned around and then I saw the girl dropping like a stone.'

A grimace of disgust contorted his face, perhaps recalling the moment of impact. He was right, when the girl toppled over the edge I had let out a yell so loud the whole of Yport must have heard.

'She didn't fall,' I told him. 'She jumped.'

The guy didn't respond. Had he grasped the difference?

'Poor girl!' the old woman on my right observed.

She was the third witness to the tragedy. I later found out that her name was Denise. Denise Joubain. Like the man in the brown jacket, she had been on the beach before me, more than a hundred metres away from the place where the girl had landed. After my frantic sprint I arrived at the body a few seconds before they did. Denise was wearing yellow socks that extended above the tops of her wellies before disappearing beneath her canvas dress and a grey coat. She was clutching a dog, a shih-tzu wearing a beige jumper with red stripes that made me think of *Where's Wally?*

'Hush now, Arnold,' she murmured into the dog's ear before continuing: 'Such a beautiful girl . . . Are you certain she jumped?'

Denise's observation struck me as idiotic.

Of course she jumped.

Then I realised I was the only one who'd witnessed the actual suicide. The other two had been strolling on the beach, looking out to sea, and had only turned their heads when I shouted.

What was she implying? That it was an accident?

In my mind's eye I saw again the terrible distress etched on that angelic face, the moment before her desperate leap.

'Positive,' I replied. 'I spoke to her up there, near the blockhouse. I tried to reason with her . . .'

As I spoke, I was aware of Denise Joubain casting a critical eye over me, as if my skin, my accent and my artificial leg were indicators I was not to be trusted.

What did she think? That it wasn't an accident? That someone had pushed her?

I craned my neck to look up the cliff, then added, as if to justify myself:

'It all happened very quickly. I got as close as I could. I tried to reach out to her. To throw her a—'

The words caught in my throat.

For the first time I noticed a detail on the body lying a metre away from me. A surreal detail . . .

Impossible!

The tragedy was replaying frame by frame in my mind.

That beautiful, despairing face.

The Burberry scarf floating from her hand.

The empty horizon.

Damn! What was I missing?

My gaze fixed on the red fabric at my feet.

There had to be a rational explanation.

There . . .

'We must do something!'

I turned. It was Denise who had spoken. For a moment I wondered whether she was addressing me or the dog clasped to her chest.

'She's right,' the man in the brown leather jacket insisted. 'We need to call the police.'

He had the voice of a heavy smoker. Above his worn leather jacket, his long straggly grey hair emerged from a bottle-green woollen cap resting on two ears that were red with cold. He struck me as someone who lived alone, divorced and unemployed. Why else would he be out here, taking stock of his life, at this time of day? He reminded me of Lanoël, the depressive maths teacher at Collège Jean-Vilar whom the students had nicknamed Xanax. In my mind, I'd already dubbed this guy on the beach Xanax, though I later discovered his name was Christian Le Medef. I did not know then that I would see him again on this same beach, the next day, almost at the same time, looking even more depressed, and that he would tell me something that would turn the pair of us into accomplices bound by the same paranoia.

Arnold, still clasped to the bosom of his mistress, carried on yapping.

Call the cops?

A tremor ran through the palm of my right hand, as if the cashmere scarf was slipping through my fingers again. My eyes no longer obeyed me, they returned to the scrap of red fabric. I must have looked ill at ease, because Denise and Xanax were eyeing me with suspicion.

Or maybe they were just waiting for me to take an initiative.

Call the cops?

Then it dawned on me that neither of them had a mobile phone. I took out my iPhone and dialled the emergency number.

'Fécamp police station,' a masculine voice replied after a few seconds.

I explained the situation. The suicide. The location. Yes, the girl was dead, there was no doubt about it, a fall of 120 metres on to the pebble beach. One witness had seen her jump, the other two had seen her hit the ground.

At the other end of the line they noted everything down. They sounded agitated, asking me to repeat the exact location, then they hung up.

'The police are on their way,' I told Denise and Xanax. 'They'll be here in ten minutes.'

They just nodded. For a while the only sound was the waves rushing over the pebbles. Xanax glanced down at his watch with every incoming wave. He didn't seem upset so much as annoyed, like when a pile-up results in a monster traffic jam and you find yourself obsessing about being late instead of thinking about the victims. I wondered why a man wandering the beach at eight in the morning would be fretting about the time.

Suddenly Denise let Arnold drop to the ground. The shih-tzu took refuge between his mistress's boots as she grabbed my arm.

'No sign of the cops! Come on, lad, give me your jacket.'

At first I couldn't work out why she was asking me to take it off, especially when it was barely five degrees out here.

'Your tracksuit top!' she demanded. 'Hand it over.'

My tracksuit? She thought my North Face WindWall windcheater was a 'tracksuit top'?

I did as she asked, and Denise used my purple windcheater to cover the girl's face and upper body.

What prompted this? Religion? Superstition? The desire to protect poor Arnold from psychological trauma?

Regardless, I was grateful to her.

As Denise arranged the makeshift shroud I took one last look at the scarf. In my head, a crazy voice was yelling:

How is this possible?

It was all I could think about. No matter how many times I ran through the sequence of events, every second, every gesture, I could come up with no coherent explanation.

The girl lying dead on the pebbles was wearing the red Burberry cashmere scarf wrapped around her neck.

4

How is this possible?

The cold bit into my bare arms. The sun, after putting in a brief appearance over the cliff above Fécamp, seemed to have dived back beneath a duvet of clouds. To warm myself up, I jogged on the spot. The temperature must have been nearing zero, but I wasn't about to ask the girl lying on the pebbles to give me back my WindWall. Besides, the cops couldn't be far away; I'd called them a good ten minutes ago. The three of us stood in silence. A few gulls mocked us from above.

Arnold, attached to his mistress by a thin leather leash, had sat down and was watching the gulls with a mixture of fear and disbelief.

Fear and disbelief.

I must have looked as stupid as the dog.

The girl lying dead on the pebbles was wearing the red Burberry cashmere scarf wrapped around her neck!

I turned it over and over inside my head, looking for a rational explanation. I was absolutely certain the girl had torn the scarf from my hands and then immediately thrown herself into the void.

I scanned the deserted sea wall, the casino car park, the thirty beach huts abandoned for the winter. Still no sign of the police.

Who could have wrapped that scarf around the corpse's neck? I had been the first to reach the body. There was no one else in the vicinity, apart from Xanax and Denise, and they'd been further away than I was. It wouldn't have been possible for them to run

23

away from the body and then make a show of approaching slowly without the slightest hint of breathlessness. Besides, why would they have done such a thing?

It made no sense.

So who else could have done it?

No one! No one could have approached the corpse on that huge deserted beach without being spotted by Denise or Xanax. They had seen the girl fall from the cliff and then walked towards her, their eyes fixed on the body . . .

My arms were shaking. From the cold. Anxiety. Fear. By a process of elimination I arrived at the one possible solution: the girl must have wrapped the scarf around her own neck as she fell!

Insane . . .

But no other explanation seemed to fit. I gauged the height of the cliff, I calculated the time it would take for a body to fall from that height. A few seconds. Three or four at most. Probably enough to wrap a scarf around your neck.

Technically, it was certainly possible.

Technically . . .

During that vertiginous fall, arms waving in the void, wind lashing at her face . . .

I watched a gull defying gravity, floating between sky and chalk.

The only way you could do that was if you'd planned the whole thing in advance, rehearsing each step over and over until you could do it without thinking, until you could set aside all emotions and fears and just focus on wrapping that damned scarf around your neck in the four seconds you have left before you hit the ground and die . . .

It made no sense.

Rehearse each step over and over? The scarf didn't even belong to the girl! I had found it by the side of the path, it had been a spur-of-the-moment decision to hold it out to her, hoping it could save her. The girl on the precipice had no way of foretelling that she would find herself clutching that piece of fabric.

My gaze drifted back to Denise and Xanax. He had lit a cigarette and she was tugging on Arnold's leash to get him out of the path of the smoke.

Keep following the process of elimination, I told myself, and you'll arrive at a solution. Let's say this girl found time, in one final reflex action, to twist that material around her throat rather than flapping her arms like a manic seagull as she fell, it still begged the question:

Why?

At that moment there was a break in the clouds and the clay-stained chalk cliffs glinted gold and silver in the sun's rays.

The police arrived minutes later. We watched as they parked their van outside the casino and set off towards us on foot. There were two of them. The younger of the two was in his forties, with a long, pebble-shaped head; he was also the slower of the two, picking his way over the pebbles and swearing whenever his fancy leather boots slipped on the wet seaweed. He looked half awake, as though he'd been called out to deal with a suicide before gulping down his first coffee of the day.

The second policeman was untroubled by the pebbles underfoot. He looked like a cop straight out of an Olivier Marchal movie, experienced, nearing retirement. His unbuttoned jacket revealed a broad torso and thick waist. He had straight, shoulder-length hair that was tied back at the base of his neck, revealing a wide forehead covered with wrinkles. Like Marlon Brando towards the end of his life.

When he came closer, my impression was confirmed.

Marlon Brando to a T.

The other cop was still ten metres away when Brando drew level with us and stood over the corpse.

'Captain Piroz,' he said in a detached tone. 'It's been a long time since we've had a suicide in these parts! Since the Normandy Bridge opened, that's been where everyone goes to throw themselves into the estuary.'

He ran both hands over his forehead as if to smooth his wrinkles, then went on:

'Do you know her?'

We all shook our heads.

'What did you see exactly?'

Xanax answered first. He described seeing the girl topple over the edge and then crash to the pebbles 120 metres below. Denise confirmed his account. I merely nodded.

'You were all here, then? No one saw what happened up there?'

Piroz stared at me as if he had registered my unease.

'Yes, I did. I was running the coastal path, as I do every morning. She was standing at the edge of the cliff, near the blockhouse. I spoke to her. I tried to stop her, but . . .'

Piroz looked down at my prosthesis, assessing whether my handicap was compatible with a daily jog.

'I . . . I go training every day,' I stammered. 'I'm an elite athlete. A Paralympian. You . . . you see.'

If he had seen, the captain didn't show it. He merely puckered his forehead, Brando-style, then bent over the corpse. He picked up my North Face jacket and placed it on the pebbles beside the body.

I hadn't been imagining it. The scarf was still wrapped around the girl's neck.

I could see nothing but that piece of fabric, but Piroz seemed oblivious to it. When he was done studying the tattered remains of her red dress, he turned his attention to the cliff, as if searching for some shrub clinging to the bare rock. Finally he turned to us.

'She couldn't have torn her dress as she fell.'

Before he could go on, I cut in:

'When I met the girl up there, her dress was already torn. Her make-up had run as well. She seemed terrified.'

Denise and Xanax were glaring at me, angry that I hadn't revealed these details before. Piroz ran a hand over his wrinkles again, as if this would stimulate the thought processes. The other cop's thoughts seemed to be miles away. His eyes were scanning the waves, the beach huts, the turbines over Fécamp. Arnold the shih-tzu seemed more concerned about the case than he was.

Piroz paid no attention to his colleague; perhaps the two of them had argued on the way here.

He knelt down among the pebbles to examine the body.

'A suicide?' he muttered between his teeth. 'You'd need a really good reason to throw yourself off a cliff . . .'

Piroz studied the torn folds of the dress.

When I looked back on it, that was moment I should have talked to the police. I should have told them the scarf was mine, in a sense; explained to them exactly what had happened up there near the blockhouse, how she'd torn that wretched piece of fabric from my hands . . .

But I said nothing. Instead I waited for a rational explanation to fall from the sky. For everything to sort itself out, for everyone to forget and move on to something else. I couldn't have predicted what Piroz was about to discover by lifting the girl's dress.

'What the hell,' the policeman whistled.

I came closer. So did Xanax and Denise.

The girl was wearing nothing under her dress.

No fuchsia lace knickers, no thong.

Purple marks ran along her thighs. Scratches, too, four of them, narrow and parallel, level with her hip, to the right of completely shaven pubes.

Denise closed her eyes and clutched Arnold to her breast again. Xanax's face had turned the colour of the tablets that he probably swallowed every morning. Pale as a ghost. My prosthesis wedged among the pebbles, and I had trouble keeping my balance.

Piroz let the dress fall back on the girl's body as if pulling the curtain over a stage.

'Christ. The kid's been raped . . . A few hours at the most. That seems a damned good reason to jump off the cliff.'

He straightened, took another look at the chalk cliff, then finally turned his eyes towards the scarf wrapped around her throat.

He untied it gently, using his fingertips.

I felt panic rising within me. Piroz had spoken of rape. My prints must be all over that scrap of material. Its fibres were drenched in my sweat, my DNA.

Too late. What could I say? Who would believe me?

Piroz ran his finger between the fabric and the girl's neck, slowly,

27

like a doctor examining a patient who has lost her voice.

'She wasn't only raped . . . she was strangled.'

In a state of shock, I replied without thinking:

'I . . . I spoke to her up there. She . . . she was alive. She jumped of her own free will. She—'

Piroz cut in: 'Your arrival probably interrupted her rapist as he was attempting to strangle her. You saved the girl's life . . . Or at least you could have . . .'

You could have?

I was troubled by his choice of words. And his version of events. It was possible a rapist might have had time to hide in the blockhouse when he heard me coming, but if that was the case, why hadn't the girl said anything? Why hadn't I noticed any marks on her neck when I reached out to her? Was it because I hadn't looked? Maybe I was too busy focusing on her face and her torn dress.

'What are you doing?' asked Denise.

Piroz was now on all fours, sniffing the skin of the corpse. Arnold was eyeing him warily. The policeman raised his head like a bloodhound tracking a scent and reported, 'Her skin smells of salt.'

I felt like I was watching a surrealist play, a group of actors improvising their lines. The second policeman, still a little way off, was looking on impassively. Perhaps it was a tactic they had developed between them. Each in his own role. One put on a show while the other observed our reactions without our noticing.

'Salt?' Xanax repeated, baffled.

'Yeah. But on this point at least there is a simple explanation.' Piroz let a long silence pass. 'The girl took a dip in the sea.'

As one, we all looked towards the Channel.

A dip? At this hour? In the middle of February? The water must be below ten degrees!

'Naked,' Piroz went on. 'Her clothes are dry.'

Denise stepped towards me. She looked as if she might faint. Without thinking, I offered her my arm.

'Skinny-dipping,' the policeman concluded. 'That may explain everything that followed. The rapist came along, saw her . . .' He combed his fingers through his hair. 'OK, time to secure the crime scene, bring in forensics and the rest of the circus. I'm going to need your names, addresses, phone numbers. Then if you could drop by the station in Fécamp this afternoon to make a statement. Hopefully by then we'll know the girl's identity.'

Denise was leaning on me with all her weight. I was openly shivering now. Piroz noticed and stared at me intently, then picked up my windcheater and handed it to me.

'I take it this belongs to you. Cover yourself up, don't catch cold, I'm going to need you.'

5

Who could believe me?

I saw the Étretat Needle right in front of me. The towering rock formation looked like a piece of a jigsaw puzzle detached from the cliff, or a monumental key that would slot into the Gate of Aval alongside it to reveal a secret cavern.

After leaving the cops on the beach, I had run for almost an hour. This was shorter than my usual run. Barely a dozen kilometres. Yport-Étretat, via the Valleuse de Vaucottes and the Brèche d'Étigues.

Time enough to empty my head. To think. To try to understand.

It couldn't have been more than three degrees, but I was drenched in sweat. The grass was slowly thawing, forming narrow streams of icy water that ran down the chalk cliffs in tiny cascades, carving ochre furrows in their wake. This seemingly eternal landscape was an illusion. The cliffs were under attack from all sides – water, ice, rain, sea – resisting, folding, yielding and dying, right before the eyes of millions of tourists who were oblivious to the resulting changes in the landscape.

The perfect crime.

I was shaking now.

I had spent the entire hour since I'd left the beach trying to make sense of it all. Captain Piroz seemed to have established a clear sequence of events. This nameless young woman comes to Yport beach, probably just as the sun is rising. She strips off her red dress and goes for a swim. Her rapist arrives, unnoticed, and watches as she gets dressed. He follows her as she climbs the coastal path, losing his scarf along the way. He corners the girl near the blockhouse, rapes her and tries to strangle her. At that moment he hears me and hides in the blockhouse before I show up. Too late.

The girl, in despair, jumps.

On the far side of the bay, a group of ramblers the size of ants were picking their way across the slippery footbridge that led to the cave they call La Chambre des Demoiselles. I looked at my watch: 11.03.

Time to go back.

My descent through the hanging valleys to Yport took less than forty-five minutes. I saw no one, apart from a lone cyclist in the Valleuse de Vaucottes and the donkey I passed by every morning on the Chemin du Couchant. There was scarcely a breeze as I climbed the last stretch of coastline to the Plaine de la Vallette. In the distance, the motionless turbines at Fécamp looked like giants on a break. Through the mist I could make out the radio mast at Yport, the blockhouse, the sheep scattered around it.

I felt a surge of anxiety.

If Piroz's theory was correct, the rapist had seen me. He had been watching me from inside the blockhouse. I was the only witness . . .

The coastal path began a gentle descent and I sped up as much as my prosthesis would allow.

The only witness.

As I passed the Rivage campsite, Yport bay exploded in the morning light. The tide was going out, revealing a lunar landscape. Emerald seaweed clung to the strewn boulders like scattered oases in a damp desert.

Following the rhythm of my limping run I hammered out another hypothesis.

What if Piroz was wrong?

What if the rapist had abandoned the girl on Yport beach after assaulting, raping, trying to strangle her? Then the girl, out of her mind, climbed the coastal path, losing her scarf along the way. Too traumatised to accept my offer of help, she jumps.

31

The steps leading to the casino echoed under my carbon prosthesis.

Whether the rape was committed on the beach or at the top of the cliff was irrelevant so far as the girl was concerned . . . But for me, these two possibilities raised a question. A question I needed to consider before Piroz started grilling me.

Did I or didn't I encounter the rapist?

Three more steps and I hopped over the casino bin bags to land on the concrete sea wall. I was outside the Sirène.

Had I encountered the rapist?

I couldn't let go of the question, until it dawned on me that there was another, more troubling question; one which Piroz was bound to pursue.

How had that damned red scarf ended up around the girl's neck? That Burberry scarf with my DNA all over it.

As I did every morning, I used the wooden balustrade of the Sirène to complete my cool-down stretches. I wasn't disturbing anyone; there were no tables outside, no chairs, and even fewer customers. To the side of the menu – €12.90 all inclusive: platter of whelks, mussels and *îles flottantes* for dessert – André had pinned up the weather forecast.

Sunshine – zero
Snow – likely above 400 metres
Temperature – approaching minus 15 degrees

At that moment, André Jozwiak appeared. He was no longer the prehistoric man who'd got up at dawn to serve my breakfast; he had taken the time to shave, comb his hair and splash on some aftershave. White shirt. Pristine jacket. Ready to welcome any Parisian tourists who showed up lost. André was what the locals call a '*horsain*' – an outsider. Before he wound up in Yport, he used to run a hotel restaurant at Bray-Dunes, the last French beach before the Belgian border. He liked to say that he had come south in search

32

of sun. And to convince the sceptics, every day he would pin up a weather forecast: the worst in France. He'd spend his evenings scouring the internet for the French town most likely to be hit by torrential rains, thunderstorms or freezing temperatures. This morning, according to the small print below the forecast, he had chosen Chaux-Neuve in the depths of the Jura mountains.

My first impulse was to tell him about the dead girl on the beach. In the fifteen years he had been landlord of the Sirène, he had got to know everyone in the village. If a woman that attractive had lived at Yport, he would certainly be able to identify her . . .

Before I could open my mouth, he came towards me holding a thick Manila envelope.

'This arrived for you, lad!'

I sat on the bed in my room: number 7, top floor, in the eaves, sea view. When I booked the Sirène, I had thought I had stumbled upon the kitschiest of hotels.

The rooms were clean and pretty. The place had recently been redecorated, sky blue with a seashell frieze, and the curtain tie-backs were made of mooring rope. Standing at the window I could see the coast all the way to the Fécamp lighthouse. Sitting on the bed, I could still make out the top of the cliffs.

My fingers trembled as I opened the envelope.

Who could be writing to me here? No one knew I was staying in Yport, apart from Ibou, Ophélie and a few other girls from the Saint Antoine Therapeutic Institute. And even then, they knew the name of the village where I was staying, but not the name of the hotel.

There was no sender's name on the envelope. Just mine, with my address, handwritten, a round, feminine hand.

Jamal Salaoui
Hôtel de la Sirène
7 Boulevard Alexandre Dumont
76111 Yport

The letter had been posted from Fécamp.

Just a few miles away.

Scraps of ochre paper fell on the bed.

The envelope contained about twenty sheets of paper. The first one leapt out at me. It was a photocopy of an article from a newspaper, *Le Courrier Cauchois* – the Fécamp edition. The headline took up the whole front page:

19-year-old found dead at the foot of the Yport cliffs

Beyond my window, the cliffs seemed to sway.

My fingers tightened on the paper. How had a local newspaper managed to get hold of this information already? The girl had jumped less than three hours ago, and the police would still be on the beach examining her corpse.

I tried to slow the manic beating of my heart, to force my eyes to focus on the sheet of paper. As I read, my breathing grew easier. I was holding in my hands an old edition of the *Courrier Cauchois*.

Very old. Almost ten years. It was dated Thursday, 10 June 2004.

What the hell!

Why send me a photocopy of a newspaper from a decade ago?

With a trembling hand, I leafed through the other pages. They all related to the same case. A nineteen-year-old girl found dead at the foot of the Yport cliffs. The envelope contained other cuttings from newspapers, local and national, as well as more confidential documents – extracts from interrogations, local police officers' notes detailing their investigation, letters exchanged between the examining magistrate and the captain in charge of the case.

As I read, the identity of the sender ceased to matter.

Everything this stranger had sent me seemed to be a factual account of events. But the events they described seemed beyond belief.

Ten years on.

6

Did I encounter the rapist?

The Morgane Avril case – Sunday, 6 June 2004

It was the first time Maxime Baron had seen a corpse. But when a group of youths ran up to him shouting, 'Officer, officer, there's a dead woman on the beach!', he had no choice but to go with them.

There was no point telling them he was only a cadet at Fécamp police station, that he wasn't actually on duty, that he was just covering for Captain Grima while he nipped out to buy some cigarettes . . .

He'd had no option but to accompany them.

The girl on Yport beach had had her skull smashed in.

She had fallen from the cliff, no doubt. Head first. Her brain was spilling out of her skull.

First Maxime threw up his breakfast on the pebbles, right in front of everyone. Then he wiped his mouth with the back of his hand and phoned his boss.

'Phil, we've got a body. On the beach. Just across from the Hôtel de la Sirène and the casino.'

Maxime looked up at the huge poster, two metres by three, stretched across the walls of the casino. A silver guitar, floating in front of the cliffs, and listed below were the names of fifteen local rock groups.

Empty cans and bottles littered the sea wall. Yport was waking up with a hangover.

Captain Philippe Grima arrived less than a minute later – long enough for Maxime to throw up again, and for a crowd to gather. Maxime doubted that his boss had any more experience of corpses than he did. His superior was barely five years older than him, and just out of Montluçon Police Academy. More of a mate than a boss. Just yesterday, after a session in the local squash club, the pair of them had sat for two hours in a seafront bar, talking football, bikes and girls. Then Grima had gone home to his wife and kid.

A five-year age gap, yet practically a lifetime separated them.

This was immediately evident: Captain Grima didn't throw up. He behaved like a boss. Instead of treating Cadet Baron like a mate, giving him a wink or a slap on the back, he issued crisp and precise orders that Maxime executed diligently. Far from taking offence at his superior officer's cool demeanour, the cadet looked to him as a role model. Could that be him in five years?

The first thing Captain Grima did was order the cadet to wipe the vomit from his chin and push back the rubberneckers. Then he took out his mobile phone and snapped about thirty photos of the scene. When this was done, he turned to the crowd of twenty or so teenagers who'd gathered and asked:

'Do any of you know this girl?'

Among them was a guy in a red waistcoat with gold buttons. He looked like a lift attendant. On his heart, above the yellow flames of the Sea View Casino logo, six letters were stitched in gold: *Jérémy*.

'I do. A girl like that isn't easy to forget. She spent the whole night at the Sea View.'

It took less than an hour to identify the girl.

Morgane Avril.

Nineteen years old.

First-year medical student.

Lived with her mother, Carmen Avril, Gîte du Dos-d'Âne, Route de Foucarmont, Neufchâtel-en-Bray.

Lieutenant Grima had no trouble reconstructing the events leading up to the tragedy. Morgane Avril had come to Yport to attend a rock festival organised by the casino: Riff on the Cliff. She was accompanied by her sister Océane and three friends: Nicolas Gravé, Clara Barthélémy and Mathieu Picard. Nicolas Gravé's Clio and its four passengers had set off from Neufchâtel-en-Bray, a hundred kilometres from Yport, at about six o'clock the previous evening. Morgane's mother had hesitated for some time before giving her daughters permission to go, even though they were adults.

Was she being overprotective? Was it apprehension? A premonition?

It was their first time at a disco. After months spent slogging away at university in Rouen, Morgane had successfully passed her first year of medical studies, coming thirty-eighth in her year. In the circumstances, it was impossible for Carmen to deny her daughter.

A preliminary examination by the medical examiner established beyond doubt the circumstances of the girl's death. Morgane Avril had been raped, between five and six in the morning, then strangled; her body was then thrown from the top of the cliff overlooking Yport.

Her face was swollen, her limbs dislocated by the impact. Her dress was torn, her underwear had been ripped off. Morgane's fuchsia thong was found the following day at the foot of the cliff, a dozen metres below the blockhouse, probably carried by the west winds. The thong bore traces of sperm and a few pubic hairs belonging to the rapist, identical to those found on Morgane's body. There was no trace, however, of the girl's handbag, despite a police search – of the Sea View cloakroom, the coastal path and the beach – that occupied three officers for two days.

During the ten hours after the discovery of Morgane Avril's corpse, Captain Grima questioned twenty-three witnesses – fifteen men and eight women – most of them locals who had spent the evening at the Sea View.

The Riff on the Cliff event had drawn almost a thousand visitors, most of whom had carried on enjoying themselves at the Sea View after the last group had finished playing. The witnesses, without exception, had been able to give an accurate description of Morgane Avril.

Beautiful.

Desirable.

Excited.

Captain Grima then spent hours rereading witness statements. Some of those questioned were clearly uncomfortable about speaking this way of a murder victim, particularly one who'd been raped, quite possibly by one of the guys who'd been checking her out in the disco, but all the witnesses – male and female – used the same terms:

Tease.

Hot.

Sexy.

They described her impromptu pole dance around one of the Sea View's oak pillars. She'd emerged from the ladies with her dress soaking wet and clinging to her breasts; she'd writhed, eel-like, on the dance floor, her hands playing with the fabric, sliding, opening, exposing her thighs, her shoulders. And all the while her gaze was locked on the men as if she were watching them through a sniper's cross hairs.

The bookish medical student letting go of her inhibitions.

No one could recall seeing Morgane after 5 a.m. No one had seen her leaving the Sea View. No one knew whether she had left alone or with someone else.

At 6 p.m. Captain Grima met with Morgane's mother, Carmen Avril. He had kept her waiting deliberately. Officially, because he was busy pursuing leads and interviewing witnesses. Unofficially, because two images were blurring in his mind: that of Morgane's shattered corpse, and that of the woman on the dance floor, desired by hundreds of men . . . and the thought of discussing this with a mother who must have been about the same age as his own unnerved him.

Carmen Avril came in. A strongbox, was Captain Grima's first impression. A strongbox that he would need to crack.

Grima took in her barrel-like figure, strapped into a suede jacket with iron buttons, her stout legs in laced boots. Carmen Avril's entire body seemed to be under lock and key, down to the thick glasses hanging from a chain around her neck and her leather handbag with its heavy metal frame. He suspected that her jacket concealed another chain, this time with a key hanging from it.

The key to her heart.

Now lost for ever, Grima thought.

The man who accompanied her looked as though he'd been labouring under a heavy burden for years. He had a thin face that ended in a pointed chin, and rubbery arms that seemed to flow along his body. Mister Tickle sprang to mind – the one with the endless arms – but Grima quickly suppressed the comparison as inappropriate in the circumstances.

An ill-matched couple, the captain thought to himself.

He indicated the two chairs in front of his desk.

'Monsieur and Madame Avril?'

'Madame,' the strongbox replied. 'Gilbert is Morgane's uncle. He's come with me.'

'And Morgane's father?'

'Morgane has no father.'

'He's . . .' the captain hesitated, running through the options. Dead. Disappeared. Gone . . .

Carmen Avril was one step ahead of him. 'Morgane never had a father . . .'

'You mean . . .' The captain had no idea what she meant, so he dragged out the pause until Carmen Avril cut in again.

'I brought her up on my own. I own a bed and breakfast, the Dos-d'Âne in Neufchâtel-en-Bray. For the last twenty-five years I've run that alone too.' She turned to her brother, her handbag rattling like a convict tugging on his chain. 'I asked Gilbert to come with me today. But usually . . .'

This time it was Grima who stepped in to finish the sentence:

'You endure life's trials alone. I understand.'

And he did understand. Carmen Avril was an almost unsinkable rock, he had grasped as much from their brief exchange, and the investigation would confirm it over the days that followed. Carmen was an institution in Neufchâtel-en-Bray. She ran a 3-star bed and breakfast renowned for its table d'hôte; she served as vice president of the community development association, responsible for tourism and culture; she'd served a term on the local council fifteen years ago. A strong, active, determined woman. No man in her life. Her brother, Gilbert Avril, was a lorry driver for a company in Gournay-en-Bray who spent half his life on the Dieppe–Newhaven ferry, transporting dairy products to England in his refrigerated truck.

'I need to know about Morgane's father,' the captain insisted. He stared at Carmen. The buttonholes of her jacket, reinforced with metal rods, reminded him of arrow slits.

She assumed a weary expression. 'Must I say it again, Captain? She has no father.'

'I have no doubt, Madame Avril, that she was brought up without a father. But from the genetic point of view, I have to know who—'

'I had IVF nineteen years ago.'

Grima took a moment to consider this. By law, in vitro fertilisation was reserved for married couples, or those who were able to show that they had lived together for at least two years.

'You have to be in a relationship for that, don't you?'

'Not in Belgium!'

So Carmen Avril really had produced two children all by herself . . . In other circumstances, Grima would probably have told her just how selfish he thought that was. Each night for the last four months he'd got up every three hours to bottle-feed his daughter Lola, five kilos of sheer wonder curled against his bare chest, and each time he thanked God that his girlfriend Sarah hadn't wanted to breast-feed.

Carmen Avril pulled on the chains of her glasses to wipe the lenses with a tissue. A little condensation, the captain thought; she's virtually in tears. He reminded himself that Carmen Avril's private life and the way she'd raised her daughter had nothing to do with Morgane's rape and murder. Fretting about the mother's psychology would only complicate matters.

'Madame Avril, I need to ask you some questions about Morgane. Intimate questions.'

In that moment he felt too young for this. Carmen was twenty years older than he was. True, he was a father, but his euphoric experience of fatherhood was limited to a few months.

'Go on.'

'Morgane was nineteen. It was her first trip to a disco. Witnesses have described her behaviour in the course of the evening as, how can I put it . . .' He pretended to search for the right term, as if this would somehow reduce the impact when he let the word drop.

'Provocative,' he said.

'Provocative?'

In Carmen's clenched hands, the armoured handbag twisted like white-hot metal. Her body swelled, but the iron bars resisted. Her glasses were like a glass dam; behind them he could see the tears welling in her eyes, betraying the pain she was trying so hard to hide.

'What do you mean by provocative?'

Grima was relying on line-of-sight sailing at this point; he knew exactly where he wanted to get to, but there was no knowing how many strokes of the oar it would take to get there.

'Desirable, Madame Avril. Attractive. Likely to catch the eye of any men present. She was aware of the way men looked at her – you know that as well as I do, Madame Avril.'

The padlock exploded. The lorry driver reached out a soft hand to calm his sister. She was seething with indignation.

'What do you mean, Captain? That Morgane deserved what happened to her? She was raped, Captain. Raped, strangled and thrown off a cliff. And you ask me if she was provocative!'

Grima thought of his own daughter, already adorable at the age of four months. How would he feel if someone told him she was provocative?

'We're on the same side, Madame Avril,' he stammered. 'We're trying to find your daughter's murderer. Every second counts. Morgane was the victim of the most heinous crime, no one is denying that. But if I am to catch her killer I must listen to what witnesses are telling me.'

'Witnesses who say my daughter was asking for it?'

Captain Grima, without knowing why, rose to his feet.

'Madame Avril, let me be clear about this, there are only two possible scenarios here. Either your daughter's murderer is a pervert, a mentally ill individual who just happened to come across Morgane that night – a random encounter in the casino car park, or on the beach, or by the light of a street lamp. If that is the case, we have almost no chance of identifying this person, because no one witnessed what happened. The second possibility is that Morgane's murderer was in the casino disco, they were on the same dance floor, he may even have talked to her. They might have left the disco together, Morgane might have gone with him of her own free will. Things took a bad turn after that, as we both know. This guy is a monster, and Morgane the most innocent victim you can imagine. But you must understand, Madame Avril, this second hypothesis significantly narrows down the list of possible suspects.'

Carmen Avril gave no reply. She loosened her grip on the leather-and-iron handbag and took out a tissue that she didn't have the energy to bring to her eyes.

Grima thought again of the witness accounts: Morgane, back arched against the oak beam, her strategically revealing dress displaying her panties and one breast. The most beautiful girl in the Sea View . . . Grima couldn't share those details with her mother. This wasn't the time or the place for that.

'Madame Avril, everyone who knew Morgane has told us that she was a good, studious, sensible girl. Going to the festival was her reward for a year of intense study . . . In your view, did Morgane attach a particular importance to that trip? A kind of . . .' Grima struggled for the appropriate euphemism '. . . *first experience* that she'd been looking forward to for a long time?'

Carmen glared at him. 'Was she determined to lose her virginity at all costs, is that what you're trying to say? Get to the point, Captain. Was she planning on giving herself to the first guy who came along, is that it?'

Grima nodded. 'She may have happened on the wrong person . . . If she was willing enough to go off with a stranger, it'll be easy to discover his identity.'

Behind the steel bars of her jacket, Madame Avril looked as if she might explode. The captain hoped a compliment might improve matters, particularly one that was sincere.

'Your daughter was pretty, Madame Avril. Very pretty. Probably the prettiest girl at the disco. Try to follow my reasoning. Morgane was spoilt for choice. Morgane was at liberty to choose the boy she wanted to go out with. If she chose her murderer rather than the other way round, we will find him. It will be easy to find him.'

Carmen Avril leapt from her chair, unleashing her fury.

'*Chose* her murderer? Did I understand correctly, Captain? You think she *chose* her murderer! Listen to me very carefully, Grima, my daughter didn't go off with anyone! My daughter was not consenting. My daughter was raped. You understand? Raped, strangled and tossed over a cliff like a dead animal.'

Philippe Grima thought again of his little Lola's warm body. Imagine raising a girl to the age of nineteen so that . . .

Yes, he understood. Of course he did. That was why he wanted to lock this guy up as fast as possible.

'I just want to find the bastard who did this to her . . .'

Mister Tickle, still sitting down, extended an arm as long as a willow branch to pull Carmen by the sleeve. Carmen stepped forward to escape her brother's hand and looked Captain Grima up and down.

'You're nothing but an incompetent young fool.'

The autopsy took place the following day.

It confirmed what they already knew. Morgane Avril was raped sometime between 5 a.m. and 6 a.m., then strangled and thrown

43

off the cliff. In that order. According to the medical examiner, she was probably dead before she was thrown over the edge. In Morgane's vagina were traces of sperm that they identified, given the chronology of events, as belonging to the rapist.

This was excellent news for Captain Grima. The next step would be to check the DNA against all the men who had attended the Riff on the Cliff festival and the Sea View, and if necessary every adult male in Yport. Several newspapers recalled the events that followed the rape and murder of English schoolgirl Caroline Dickinson in 1996 while on a school trip to Brittany. All the men in Pleine-Fougères had to give DNA samples for testing . . . then all possible suspects in Brittany and beyond – more than 3,500 people. Eight years on, would a judge have the guts to initiate testing on this scale in Normandy?

The autopsy revealed two additional details, both of which reinforced Captain Grima's hypothesis.

First, Morgane Avril, before being killed and raped, had taken a dip in the sea. Naked. The medical examiners were categorical: the traces of salt and iodine left no room for doubt. She had swum in the sea, and then she had put her dress back on. This occurred before she was raped. For Captain Grima, it was as if another piece of the puzzle had fallen into place. Morgane follows a stranger she has picked up at the Sea View. She takes it up a level with a midnight skinny-dip for the pair of them, far from prying eyes. Then the adventure turns to tragedy. Morgane gets dressed, decides to leave things there, gives the stranger a parting kiss – and he loses control.

The second detail was even stranger. The rapist hadn't strangled Morgane Avril with his hands, but with a scarf. The autopsy findings were very precise: the red cashmere fibres taken from the victim's neck were of exceptional quality and sufficiently rare that the experts were able to identify the garment they came from: a Burberry scarf.

Four hundred and twenty-five euros for a piece of fabric.

A red scarf . . .

Captain Grima had whistled between his teeth.

The noose would soon be tightening around the rapist. There couldn't be many young people in Yport who wore a scarf like that around their necks.

I read every single one of the pages a second time: the newspaper articles, the police reports, all the details of the investigation recorded by Captain Grima.

A nineteen-year-old girl, raped, strangled and thrown from the top of the cliff overlooking Yport.
Almost ten years ago. June 2004.
After taking a dip in the sea, naked.
Strangled with a red cashmere Burberry scarf.

The room seemed to be spinning around me. My laptop was on the table. Connected.

I feverishly typed a few keywords into a search engine.

Morgane Avril. Rape. Yport.

Google took a nanosecond to deliver the results: dozens of articles devoted to the Morgane Avril case. I skimmed the summaries. They confirmed that the pages I'd been sent were accurate to the last detail.

I stood up. Through the window, the cliffs taunted me. Sheep grazed calmly around the blockhouse, as if this morning's drama had never taken place. As if I had dreamed that scene, a scene that had happened not a few hours ago, but ten years ago.

I was going mad.

I picked up the envelope again and ran my finger over the postmark.

Fécamp
5.43 p.m.
18.02.14
France

45

Someone had posted this package, from Fécamp, yesterday! Someone who knew I was going to meet that girl on the cliff the following day. Someone who also knew that this girl would die in the same way as another had died, ten years previously, with one exception . . . This one hadn't been thrown to her death from the top of the cliff, like Morgane Avril. She had jumped, alive, and of her own free will.

It made no sense.

Who could have guessed? How? Why?

I looked at the pristine bed, the pillows plumped nicely against the sky-blue wallpaper of the room.

No, I hadn't been dreaming! Quite the contrary. The green LED display of the alarm clock reminded me as if delivering a command: 12.53.

It was time to catch the 1.15 p.m. bus that would take me to Fécamp for my meeting with Piroz.

7

Strangled with a red cashmere Burberry scarf?

I climbed the three steps to the door of Fécamp police station. At reception, a girl with eyes as blue as the colour of her blouse gave me an air-hostess smile.

'I have an appointment with Captain Piroz.'

She had a mermaid's voice, to lure all the local unemployed into the nets of the police: 'Last door on the right, you can't miss it, it's got his name on it.'

I walked through a cluttered hallway that housed a photocopier and several filing cabinets creaking under stacks of files. The walls were lined with recruitment posters. I continued down a long corridor. Uniformed men were busy behind computers. Chairs were lined up near the doors.

Xanax was sitting twenty metres ahead of me. He was wearing the same leather jacket as he had worn this morning. I sat down next to him. He smiled at me, or at least more than he had done earlier.

'Denise is already in there,' he said. 'Arnold too . . . After that it's my turn.'

I returned his smile and then we didn't say another word. I tried to remember his real name, the one he had given to the police this morning. It came back to me after a few minutes. Le Medef. Christian Le Medef. Ironic that someone who matched the stereotype of a victim of the system should have the same name as the French bosses' organisation.

We waited. All that was missing was a coffee table, *Le Figaro* and *Paris Match*. I was tempted to get my iPhone out and search the internet for more information about the Morgane Avril case. I didn't know who had sent the package of cuttings to the Sirène, but the police must surely have noticed the many points this case had in common with the 2004 one.

The red-scarf rapist was back, ten years on.

Xanax kept looking at his watch in annoyance. The police were coming and going, up and down the corridor. Further on, at the coffee machine, a woman was getting annoyed because every time she put her a coin in the slot, it was rejected. She was wearing tight jeans that showed off her figure, and her red hair was tied in a ponytail that cascaded down her neck. I was intrigued. Who wore ponytails these days? I waited impatiently for her to turn around so that I could see her face.

No such luck! She still had her back turned when the door to Piroz's office opened and Denise came out, with Arnold wedged under her arm. He was the witness to the tragedy who had changed his outfit; he was now wearing an elegant red and blue Fair Isle sweater, almost in the colours of the gendarmerie. Piroz came out with her and shook her hand.

'Monsieur Le Medef, you're next . . .'

Xanax and Piroz disappeared through the door, which the captain closed behind them. Denise, stroking Arnold like a frail child who had just been to see the doctor, stared at me with clear eyes.

'You're in for a wait – he'll be at least a quarter of an hour. They want to know everything, even the things we didn't see.'

Denise's wrinkled hands disappeared into the coat of her shih-tzu, all the while shifting from one leg to the other as if she urgently needed to go for a wee.

Or perhaps she was just anxious to talk to me.

She leaned towards me, slowly, glancing out of the corner of her eye at the policemen coming and going.

'Young man, I must apologise. I was obliged to tell them the truth.'

The truth?

'What truth?' I asked, stunned.

Denise leaned forward again.

'You remember, this morning, you told the policeman that we saw the girl jump. All three of us. They were very insistent on that point. So I was obliged to clarify.'

She adjusted Arnold's pullover while a policeman passed in front of us, then continued in a low voice:

'I didn't see her jump. I saw the girl fall, I saw her land on the pebbles, and I'm sure the same is true of the gentleman who is with the captain now. But I didn't see her jump! Besides, from where we were standing, we couldn't see what was happening up above – the policemen checked.'

She was looking at me as if I were a Jew she had denounced to the Gestapo, with the faux apologetic look of a decent woman who was only doing her duty.

'You must understand, there was nothing else I could have done.'

I adopted the demeanour of a docile young man and gave her the response she was hoping for: 'Of course. No problem. Don't worry, the investigation won't go on too long, it was . . . it was a suicide.'

Denise straightened and looked at me, almost incredulous, as if I were the most naive man on earth. At last she set Arnold down on the floor and walked away. The shih-tzu followed her, sniffing each office door like an amateur sleuth delighted to visit the lair of the professionals.

I stretched out my prosthetic leg. My mind was in chaos.

In front of me, the red-haired girl had finally triumphed over the drinks machine. She turned, smiling. Her gaze met mine for a fraction of a second, without dropping below my knee. That was rare, probably as rare as a boy looking at a girl without his eyes plummeting to her chest.

She passed me, plastic cup in hand, then disappeared around the corner. She was rather cute, with her ponytail and her face sprinkled with freckles. The kind of cheeky face that would drive the cops crazy.

*

'Monsieur Salaoui?'

A good twenty minutes had passed since Xanax had gone inside. We passed in the doorway without a word, then I went into Captain Piroz's office.

'Sit down, Monsieur Salaoui.'

I did as he asked. In front of me, a huge model sailing boat stood on Piroz's desk, a three-master mounted on a mahogany stand.

The captain cleared his throat. 'It's a scale model of the *Étoile-de-Noël*! Built in Dundee, 1920, one of the last Newfoundland fishing vessels to sail out of Fécamp before the Second World War. It belonged to my great grandfather!'

Had Piroz built this model himself?

When I was a kid, my mother's colleagues in the canteen where she worked gave me a Meccano model for Christmas. A fifteen-centimetre motorbike that moved if you picked it up between your thumb and index finger and made it roll along the carpet. Big deal! I may have been only twelve years old but I was already working on my cousin Latif's Yamaha VMAX every weekend.

'Three hundred hours, that took!' Piroz went on. 'The fishery museum commissioned another one, *Le Dauphin*, the last trawler out of Fécamp. Everyone in town wept over that boat, but they will have to wait – I can't make a start on the model until I retire. Less than a year to go – they can hold out that long, right?'

Unsure what he expected me to say to his, I nodded. Piroz brushed back his hair with the palm of his hand.

'You don't give a damn about my models, do you, Salaoui? This old cop's a bit of a fool, that's what you're thinking, isn't it?'

I didn't bother to answer. I waited to see if Piroz was going to come up with a smart riposte. Files were stacked up on his desk behind the Newfoundland fishing vessel. I couldn't read the name written on the bottle-green dossier on top.

The wrinkles on Piroz's forehead lengthened.

'This isn't a suicide, Monsieur Salaoui.'

The information hit me like a slap in the face. Piroz had a sense of timing, he didn't give me time to draw breath before continuing:

'We've identified the victim.'

He opened the file and held out a sheet of paper.

'Here you go, Salaoui, after all, it's not confidential.'

I looked at it: both sides of an identity card, photocopied on a single page.

Magali Verron
b. 21 January 1995, Charlesbourg, Québec
Height: 1.73 m
Distinguishing features: none

I registered the information.

'I'm sorry, Captain. I've never heard of her.'

Piroz didn't seem to care what I had to say; he carried on reading from the file:

'She was a rep for a large pharmaceutical company. Yesterday she met about ten doctors from Fécamp and Criquetot-l'Esneval. According to her diary, she was due to see more. She probably spent the night in Yport or nearby, but for now we have no record of her having stayed in any of the local hotels.'

Piroz turned the page and then looked up from his file as if to check that I was paying attention.

'On the other hand, the sequence of events since this morning is quite clear. Magali Verron went for a swim in the sea at around five in the morning. She was raped sometime before six, the medical examiners are quite clear about that. They found traces of sperm in her vagina, bruises on her skin. Her dress was torn, but her panties – a thong, presumably fuchsia to match her bra – have yet to be found. We're still looking. Same goes for her handbag. Not a trace.'

Piroz's words reverberated in my head.

He had to have made the connection with the murder of Morgane Avril ten years before. All the details corresponded. The rape. The place and time of the attack. The age of the victim. The naked early morning swim. The missing panties.

Except for her death . . .

I cleared my throat to speak, to bring up the subject of the Avril case, but Captain Piroz waved his hand to indicate that he hadn't finished.

'After being raped, Magali Verron was strangled.' He paused for a long time. 'With the scarf that we found wrapped around her neck. You remember? A cashmere scarf, in a red tartan pattern. A Burberry scarf – and those things cost a small fortune. If I told you how much, Salaoui, you wouldn't believe it!

8

Would you believe it?

Captain Piroz moistened his finger with his tongue and ran it over the varnished hull of the *Étoile-de-Noël* to remove an invisible mark.

I didn't ask him to repeat himself.

I didn't ask him if he was sure the medical examiners knew what they were doing, how they could possibly claim that Magali Verron had been strangled with that red scarf before falling off the cliff.

I didn't say anything that might have aroused his suspicions. Instead I remained silent, replaying this morning's events in my mind. The Burberry scarf caught on the barbed wire on the hiking path, my hand hesitating, then pulling it away, the same hand tossing it to Magali, Magali's hand catching it, pulling it, tugging it from my grasp. The same girl, 120 metres and four seconds down below, with the scarf wrapped around her neck.

Tell him about it!

A voice in the depths of my head gave me an order.

Tell him about the scarf! Tell him everything! The rapist's prints are probably on that scrap of fabric, but so are yours. The police are bound to find them anyway . . .

'Captain Piroz . . .'

What should I say?

That Magali had wrapped the scarf around her neck as she threw herself off the cliff? Reveal that I was the last one to touch that scrap of fabric? That would be tantamount to accusing myself. Of rape. Of murder. I'd be totally screwed.

53

'Yes, Monsieur Salaoui?' Piroz's wrinkled face showed as much sign of brain activity as a flatlining encephalogram.

'I . . .'

I had hesitated too long before taking the plunge. My head filled with reasons to remain silent: Piroz said they had found traces of the rapist's sperm, so the investigators would have his DNA within a week – and it would probably be a match for Morgane Avril's killer. Then I would be cleared. Then would be time to tell my own version.

Having made up my mind, I decided to change tactics and go on the attack.

'I have a question for you, Captain Piroz. Don't you think that this case bears a striking similarity to the Morgane Avril case? Yport, June 2004. Surely you recall the investigation?'

Piroz was visibly shaken. This was probably the last thing he'd expected to hear, but he parried my question:

'You remember that case, Monsieur Salaoui?'

Now it was my turn to be caught off guard. I couldn't tell him about the mail I had received, not yet.

'Ten years ago, but it's all the locals talk about. Coincidences like that are hard to ignore, don't you agree? The rape, the naked swim in the sea, the torn red dress . . .'

I paused a moment too long.

'The red cashmere scarf,' Piroz finished for me. 'Same murder weapon for both crimes . . .' He stared me straight in the eye. 'You can rest assured, Monsieur Salaoui, we are aware of the similarities with the Morgane Avril case. But as you know, that murder took place ten years ago . . . Right now, if you don't mind, let's focus on the murder of Magali Verron.'

Piroz turned to a new page of his file, as if to give me time to think. I dived in as quickly as I could:

'Magali was alive when I met her on the clifftop. I must have disturbed her rapist, he didn't have time to strangle her. Not completely . . .'

The captain looked at me for a long time. His forehead wrinkled into a V, forming an arrow pointing at the report in front of him.

'The medical examiner takes a different view, Monsieur Salaoui. The results of the autopsy show that Magali was asphyxiated and then thrown over the edge . . .'

Piroz forced a smile before continuing:

'But there is, I grant you, one area of doubt, a discrepancy of a few minutes. We'll talk about that another time, once the details have been confirmed. In the meantime, Monsieur Salaoui, I want you to talk me through your encounter with Magali Verron this morning.'

The captain recorded every detail. The exact location. The torn dress. The few words Magali said to me:

Don't come any closer.
If you take so much as a step, I'll jump . . .
You could never understand. Keep running.
Go! Get out of here, now!

I described the look on Magali's face, every move she made.

It took more than ten minutes for Piroz to note it all down.

'Good. Very good, Monsieur Salaoui.'

He leaned forward and, with the tip of his index finger, adjusted the five-millimetre pilot at the helm of the *Étoile-de-Noël* so that he was no longer leaning to one side.

'Now, if you don't mind, let's talk about you.'

He opened his green folder. On the first page I saw the logo of the Saint Antoine Therapeutic Institute.

Damn!

Piroz went for the jugular.

'You work in an asylum, Monsieur Salaoui?'

'No, Captain. The Saint Antoine is a therapeutic and educational facility. Our students aren't insane, they're just young people with physical and behavioural disorders.'

'Are you part of the educational staff?'

'No, Captain.'

'The therapeutic side of things?'

'No, I'm responsible for maintenance. Vehicles, carpentry, plumbing, anything that needs fixing. The facility is eight hundred square metres in area, with a garden three times that, and a fleet of six Citroën vans.'

The captain had stopped taking notes; he wasn't interested in my duties.

'Have you been at the Saint Antoine Institute for long?'

Have you been there, not *have you worked there.* I knew exactly what he was insinuating and I'd had enough of his games. My prosthesis scraped the floor as I shifted in my chair.

'Let me spell it out for you, Captain. I didn't spend my childhood in the Institute. I wasn't some insane inmate who was kept on because the staff didn't know what else to do with him when he turned eighteen. I am a qualified building maintenance officer. They hired me six years ago.'

Piroz blew in the direction of the ship's mast as if to get rid of a speck of dust. For a moment he watched the paper sails swell, then immersed himself in the file again.

'Here we go: recruited in 2008 as part of a drive to get more disabled employees on the payroll. Your employers have given me all the details.'

This bastard was out to get me. I could tell from his attitude which parts of my CV had leapt out at him as they'd been highlighted with a neon marker.

Jamal Salaoui.

Arab. Disabled. Works with mad kids . . .

Ideal profile for a rapist.

Mentally I added a new category to my list of everyday torturers: vicious gods, sadistic teachers, fascist little bosses, bigoted cops . . .

'Monsieur Salaoui, we've been in contact with your immediate superior, Monsieur Jérôme Pinelli.'

'He's on holiday!'

For the first time Piroz almost cracked a smile, revealing his yellowing teeth.

'I got through to him in Courchevel. He was in the ski lift on his way to the Jockeys black piste. He confirmed it.'

What did he confirm? I seethed, waiting for him to elaborate.

'Your identity, Monsieur Salaoui. Your role at the Saint Antoine

Institute. One point in your favour, you don't have a criminal record – you couldn't work with special needs youngsters if you didn't have a clean record. Having said that . . .'

I suppressed the urge to send all the miniature figures on the deck of the *Étoile-de-Noël* into orbit with a flick of my fingers.

'What?'

'Jérôme Pinelli has expressed reservations.'

What had that arsehole been saying now?

'Reservations?'

'He was telling me about Ophélie Parodi. A fifteen-year-old girl who has spent the last eighteen months at the Institute.'

Two-faced bastard! Sitting on his ski lift, making accusations. He and Piroz must have hit it off straight away.

'He implied that you were very close to little Ophélie, much too close, according to the psychologists at the Institute. You were reprimanded about it several times . . .'

Maybe instead of aiming a flick of the fingers at those miniature sailors I should crush all three masts with my fist, just for the pleasure of seeing Piroz's reaction.

But I remained surprisingly calm. Soothed, perhaps, by the thought of Ophélie.

'You need to check your sources, Captain. An office manager isn't always best placed to comment. Many of my colleagues would take a very different view to Jérôme Pinelli. But . . . I don't understand what my job at the Institute has to do with the death of Magali Verron. Let's get to the point, Captain. Am I being accused of pushing that girl off the cliff? Of raping her?'

Piroz slowly ran his hand over his hair. That bastard had been waiting for a reaction from me. He took his time closing the green file, making me wait for his response.

'Take it easy, Monsieur Salaoui. For the moment, you are the chief witness in a case that is turning out to be very complicated. You are the only one who saw Magali Verron jump of her own free will. The only one to suggest it was suicide, despite the findings of the medical examiner . . .'

'"For the moment"?'

'To be frank, Monsieur Salaoui, given the evidence at my disposal, I could take you into custody right now.'

I fell back into my chair, stunned.

'You're a fast runner, Monsieur Salaoui, even on one leg – it's in your file. If you're the rapist and I let you go . . .'

Piroz felt that he had seized the advantage. He wasn't holding back.

'So before you go accusing me of harassment, Monsieur Salaoui, you should think very carefully. I'm going to take a chance and let you remain at liberty until the DNA results are in. I'll see you again tomorrow, 2 p.m., in this office.'

With that he sprang to his feet, picked up the green file, and then walked around the desk to stand behind me.

'What happened to you, Monsieur Salaoui?'

'What do you mean?'

'Your leg.'

I didn't like the way he was looking at me.

On Piroz's desk, a loose sheet was lying on top of a stack of files. It was blank apart from a table made up of eight numbers arranged in four squares:

2/2	3/0
0/3	1/1

I was intrigued. Was it some kind of brain-teaser? Was Piroz filling the remaining months until his retirement with sudoku puzzles?'

'You haven't answered my question, Monsieur Salaoui.'

I had to crane my neck to speak to him.

'A mistake, Captain. A policeman shot at me. I was making my getaway after robbing the BNP, Rue Soufflot, in the fifth arrondissement. I was a fast runner in those days, but not fast enough. I got away with it because I was wearing a Betty Boop mask so they couldn't identify me . . .'

'Are you taking the piss?'

'I'm playing it down.'

Piroz shrugged, stepped forward and opened a drawer.

'While we're on the subject of Betty Boop . . .'

He tossed an old copy of *Playboy* into my lap.

'Go next door and fill a sample jar for me.'

'With sperm?'

'What do you think? Crème Chantilly? Yes, with sperm.'

Piroz's request struck me as almost surreal.

'Is this the normal procedure?'

'What's the problem? You want me to hold it for you?'

'And if I refuse?'

The captain sighed. 'Surely it's not in your interest to refuse, Salaoui – unless that's your sperm in Magali Verron's vagina? And before you go, I'm also going to need fingernail and hair samples from you for DNA testing.'

I rolled up the *Playboy* and got to my feet. He was right. I was blameless. Everything would be much simpler once they had compared my DNA with the rapist's. Then I would make Piroz, Pinelli and all the others eat their words . . .

At least, that was what I thought.

How could I have thought otherwise?

My sperm, my hair, my fingernails . . .

None of them had been in contact with that girl.

Since then, I've thought a lot about the expression on Denise's face when I told her about Morgane Avril's suicide. As if she couldn't believe I could be so naive . . .

She was right.

Naive.

Being innocent, having harmed no one, being blameless – it isn't enough.

No smoke without fire. Forget proof, forget the truth, doubt always creeps in.

In spite of everything.

In spite of you?

59

Because, on second thoughts, isn't it easier to believe the cops and the forensic experts rather than a disabled Arab who works with crazy kids?

9

No smoke without fire?

'It doesn't take five-cent coins . . . It swallows twenty-cent coins – I've tried. It will only accept one-euro coins, and it doesn't give change,' said a woman's voice behind me.

I gave up on the drinks machine and turned to face her.

'The cops are all crooks,' she added.

It was the red-haired girl. She smiled at me, her pink lips slightly parted over milky teeth. With her bright black eyes and little turned-up nose, she reminded me of a shrew. All she needed was some fine nylon whiskers protruding from the freckles on her cheeks.

I returned her smile. 'Too right,' I said.

Following her advice, I put in a one-euro coin and selected an Americano without sugar. She held out her plastic cup. I tapped mine against it.

'They've kept me waiting for forty-five minutes. What about you?'

'I've finished . . . For today, at least. But I think I'm going to have to take out a season ticket . . .'

I watched as she lapped at her drink with a little pink tongue. It called to mind the calendars my mother would hang over the kitchen sink every year, with pictures of kittens drinking from bowls of milk, girls in tutus around a piano. My first erotic photographs.

The girl looked at me curiously.

'What are you here for?'

61

I hesitated for a second, barely more than that.

'I'm a witness. A girl threw herself off Yport cliff. I was there right before she jumped, but there was nothing I could do.'

She pursed her lips. Her mousy eyes clouded.

'That's awful. Do they . . . do they know why she did it?'

'They have their suspicions. According to the investigation, she was raped just before she committed suicide. The rapist tried to strangle her as well.'

'My God . . .'

The little shrew put a hand over her incisors, as if frightened, then immediately recovered. She obviously enjoyed play-acting.

'At least you're not the rapist?'

It was the kind of no-holds-barred repartee I shared with Ibou. I loved that blend of mischief and black humour.

'No, I don't think so. We'll soon find out, I've just given the policeman my sperm . . .'

She paused for a moment, as if imagining the scene in her head: a guy masturbating behind the curtain of the office next door, then studied me intently, her eyes dropping to my crotch without apparently noticing my artificial leg.

Hats off, mademoiselle! But I was sure it was my disability that had attracted her. The fact I was different. She was the kind of girl who was drawn to anything that deviated from the norm. She stared at me with her deep black pupils.

'Well that's good news! If you are the rapist, I needn't worry about you for a few minutes at least. The beast is sated.'

I checked my watch. 'Don't underestimate me . . . Being sexually attacked in a police station would add a bit of spice, don't you think?'

I burst out laughing, but the little shrew wasn't quite as brave as she let on. Her little white teeth attacked the plastic rim of the cup. Before she tore a hole in it, I went on:

'What about you?'

'Me?'

'Why have the cops kept you waiting forty-five minutes?'

By way of reply, she reached into the back pocket of her jeans and pulled out a crumpled piece of paper.

'I'm waiting for them to rubber-stamp this so I can collect pebbles from the beach.'

'I'm sorry?'

She burst out laughing. 'My turn to surprise you!'

She held out her hand. 'Mona Salinas. I may not look it, but I'm a boring postdoctoral fellow in experimental chemistry. I have a grant funded by P@nshee Computer Techonologies, an Indo-American multinational specialising in electronic components for the computer industry . . .'

'What does that have to do with pebbles?'

She twisted the cup between her fingers. I wondered if she was nervous because of what I'd been saying about rape.

'I'll let you guess . . .' she taunted.

The connection between computers and pebbles? No idea.

Still, I pretended to be thinking. Oddly enough, I liked studious girls, the swats who were always top of the class. Most of the guys I hung out with in La Courneuve avoided them like the plague . . . Not me. I'd found that, once you got to know them, they were the most fun. And the least stuck-up. Mind you, it wasn't often I got to talk to a girl who was a postdoctoral fellow in experimental chemistry.

My little mouse was growing impatient.

'Cat got your tongue?'

I nodded apologetically.

'OK!' she said. 'I'll try to keep it short. Silicium is an essential component in the manufacture of computers. It's a semiconductor, used in computer chips You've heard of Silicon Valley in the United States? That's where the name comes from, silicium, not from the gelatinous breasts of Californian women.'

Inevitably, my eyes darted for a quarter of a second to her pert little breasts, white and sprinkled with freckles. Milk and honey.

Like a tightrope walker, I miraculously regained my balance on the thread of our conversation.

'I must be an idiot, but I still don't see what that has to do with your pebbles.'

63

She was amused by my puzzlement.

'Patience. I'm getting there. Silicon, silicium, if you're still following me, only appears in a single compact form in the natural state: pebbles! And English Channel pebbles have the highest level of silicon in the world.'

'Really?'

'Scientifically proven. Today, the world capital of pebbles is Cayeux-sur-Mer, in Picardy. But here in Normandy they claim their pebbles are even purer. The largest reserves of silicon in the world, both in terms of quality and quantity.'

I thought of those endless grey pebbles washed by the waves, to the general indifference of passers-by. It was hard to believe they constituted a high-tech treasure trove.

'And you need permission from the police to collect pebbles?'

'Yes! A century ago they used thousands of tons to build the local roads, houses and churches. But since then they've realised that the pebbles protect the cliffs, and everything built on top of them. So nowadays collection is strictly forbidden, unless you manage to obtain authorisation.'

'Because you work for a big Indo-American multinational that might invest in the region, for example.'

'You've got it. And I only take a few hundred pebbles. To give you an idea, the silicium used in electronics needs to be 99.9999999 per cent pure.' Her mouth formed the 9s as if she were blowing little soap bubbles. 'That's the current standard, but P@nshee, my company, wants another two or three 9s. It's my job to find out if we can gain a few extra 9s after the decimal point thanks to the pebbles of Fécamp, Yport or Étretat.'

'And you've got your chemistry set with you?'

'Yes! A hammer, pliers, test tubes, a microscope and a laptop crammed with complicated software . . .'

I wanted to stay with her. I didn't understand everything she was telling me – for all I knew, she was having me on with her talk of silicon and nine figures after the decimal point – but I liked it all the same! I loved the idea that something as stupid as a pebble might contain some unique treasure.

We both emptied our cups in silence. I was leaving it to Mona to decide if she wanted to pursue this. All she had to do was ask my name and what I was doing in Yport, and I would take out the flyer for the Mont Blanc Ultra-Trail and tell her of the record-breaking feat I was planning.

The silence continued.

I threw my cup into the bin. Bullseye!

She did the same. Equaliser.

I realised that Mona wasn't planning to take it further.

'Delighted to have met you, Mona. Maybe I'll see you again tomorrow, if you're still waiting for your application to be rubber-stamped when they bring me back in handcuffs . . .'

She rested a hand on my shoulder and drew close to my ear, murmuring:

'My little antennae tell me we'll see one another before tomorrow.'

I said nothing, content to enjoy the gentle pressure of her palm. She loved speaking in riddles, and I hadn't a clue what they meant.

'My antennae are powerful. They also tell me that you're staying in Yport. Hôtel de la Sirène. Room number 7.'

She had said too much. I wondered if she had been sent to spy on me. Perhaps Piroz was the cat and she was the mouse.

'How do you know that?'

She leaned forward again. Her orange-painted fingernails brushed my shoulder blade.

'My antennae! Poor defenceless creatures like me need to be well informed if they're to survive encounters with predators of your kind.'

She stood up abruptly and looked at her watch.

'Thirteen minutes! I'm going to have to leave you. Any minute now the beast will awake , and I'll no longer be safe in your company.'

'I'm not going to devour you here, not bang in the middle of the police station.'

'Maybe not here. But later?'

Later?

It didn't look as though Mona wanted to help me understand.

She took three steps towards the corridor and walked towards one of the offices.

'Sorry to abandon you, but I really need to get one of these cops to approve this for me.'

'Good luck, then.'

I was about to set off in the direction of the exit when Mona paused in the doorway to one of the offices and said:

'See you this evening! Don't be late.'

10

See you this evening?

The bus dropped me in Yport, Place Jean-Paul Laurens, before continuing on towards Le Havre. Only a fifteen-minute journey, but a wait of almost three quarters of an hour in Fécamp. I had time to think again about Piroz's investigation. I felt almost relieved. The rapist's sperm, his prints, those coincidences with the Morgane Avril murder ten years ago, all proved (or would prove) that I had nothing to do with it.

I avoided thinking about the shadowy areas . . .

They would brighten. Like the twilight sun whose last rays were fraying the clouds into rainbow lace. The famous light of the Impressionists – I couldn't help recognising it, even though I'd never set foot in a museum; Yport was worth the detour just for that.

I set off towards the sea, thoughts of Mona running through my mind. Her face followed me like a watermark superimposed over the sunset. It lacked the tragic grace of Magali Verron, her desperate beauty, that thing that cuts through your heart like a blade. No . . . Mona was someone you'd want to share a beer with, a mate of the opposite sex. The sort of mate you'd share a bed with too, and it would be no more complicated than sharing a beer. Perhaps that was love.

Love from the male perspective.

As far as I knew.

I passed a butcher's shop. Behind the glass the proprietor was giving me a sidelong glance, as if I might knock her pavement out of shape by walking on it with my artificial leg.

Bitch!

Mona's face drove the butcher from my mind. Why had she taken an interest in me?

Why had she approached me?

Because there was nothing more natural in the world between a man and a woman lost in a place where they are more or less the only strangers of the same age? Probably. I had never been able to shake that feeling of inferiority; guilt, almost. How could a girl be interested in me without my having to develop a strategy to win her over? There were so many guys out there who would make a better catch than me . . .

I stepped off the pavement to make way for two old ladies who were coming in the opposite direction, walking sticks in their fists, more disabled than me.

In February, Yport was like an old people's home, a pretty convalescent hospital beside the sea. You might even say that the town itself was an old lady. A grandmother you would only visit when the weather was fine, in the holidays, bringing the children along to fill gaps in the conversation and make some noise. A grandmother who owned a big garden with weeds and swings that rusted all year.

Yport reminded me of Djamila, my grandmother. Not because she lived beside the sea, somewhere like Essaouira or Agadir, far from it! She lived in Drancy, the Géricault Tower, beyond the ring road, but her sixth-floor flat overlooked a big public garden. When I was a kid I used to go there with my cousins, and the playground of Tower B was our Adventureland. The last time I dropped by, the playground was still there – the pony on a spring, the monkey bridge – but the place was empty apart from a few old people sitting on benches with no kids to keep an eye on. Any child that wandered in would have found themselves put on display like some exotic animal in a zoo for the retired.

I carried on along the seafront. There was a stiff breeze coming off the sea. Another twenty metres and I had reached the Sirène.

Mona brought back memories of my childhood, although I couldn't think why.

As soon as I entered the hotel, André Jozwiak stepped out to greet me, all smiles.

An envelope in his hand.

I put out a hand to steady myself, as if clutching the fishermen's ropes that decorated the plaster moulding. I could make out the UPS stamp on the parcel. A courier must have dropped the package off this afternoon. André was amused.

'For someone who never used to receive any mail . . . Have you written a manuscript and all the publishing houses are rejecting you?'

He held out the envelope. My name was written on the front in sky-blue ink; the same handwriting as this morning's package.

'. . . Or you've got a new girlfriend and your exes are sending your love letters back?' André went on.

I grabbed the parcel and headed for the stairs leading up to my room.

'Thanks, André.'

'Proofs to correct?' he carried on, undeterred. 'You've got your teacher-training certificate and schools in deprived areas want to use their government funding to hire you?'

Clearly he wasn't going to stop unless he got an answer, so I gave him one:

'They're mail order catalogues. Medical journals. Nothing but pictures of artificial left feet.'

The landlord's laughter echoed around the stairwell.

'Dinner's at seven,' he called after me.

The contents of the envelope were spread across the bed.

Like this morning's package, it contained newspaper articles, Captain Grima's case notes, statements from witnesses, all relating to the Morgane Avril case. This anonymous sender was certainly the master of suspense . . .

I spread out the sheets of paper and sat down to read. If my mysterious correspondent was so intent on arousing my curiosity, I wasn't about to deprive him of his pleasure.

Morgane Avril case – June 2004

In spite of his youth and lack of experience, Captain Philippe Grima had shown himself to be a remarkably efficient police officer. Less than three days after the murder of Morgane Avril, ninety per cent of the male population of Yport between the ages of fifteen and seventy-five had agreed to provide DNA samples. Of the young men who had attended the Riff on the Cliff, just over seventy per cent provided sperm for testing (323 samples, to be precise). None of the samples were a match for the rapist's DNA.

Though Captain Grima soon realised this time-consuming exercise would achieve nothing, Judge Nadeau-Loquet insisted that, by eliminating most of the population from the inquiry, they were tightening the net on the perpetrator.

In the meantime Captain Grima continued to question the main witnesses, including those whose DNA had ruled them out as suspects. At first he spent twelve-hour days at the station and nights at home with a reheated meal on one knee and little Lola's head on the other. He'd end up falling asleep either in front of the last witnesses or in the arms of his four-month-old daughter. His wife, Sarah, threw him out for the duration of the investigation, so from 21 June to 12 July 2004 he spent three weeks sleeping on a camp bed in the station cafeteria, calling in on his family every third day with a bag of croissants.

Gradually the investigation pieced together the events leading up to Morgane Avril's death. Although she was nineteen, for Morgane that evening, 5 June 2004, was her first real night out. Her mother, Carmen, had only given her consent to the trip because the driver of the Clio, twenty-four-year-old Nicolas Gravé, who was in his final year of forestry management studies at Mesnières-en-Bray, would be there to keep an eye on Morgane and her other daughter, Océane. She also considered the other two passengers – Clara Barthélémy, nineteen, a teaching assistant at Charles Perrault kindergarten in Neufchâtel, and Mathieu Picard, twenty-one, a medical student like Morgane, but already in his third year – to be trustworthy.

They had left Neufchâtel-en-Bray at about 6 p.m., and arrived in Yport just over an hour later. They ate kebabs on the beach, sitting on the pebbles in front of the casino like hundreds of other young festival-goers, then attended the Riff on the Cliff concert. There was a party atmosphere, but nothing over the top. Morgane was excited, but no more than anyone else.

The headline act, local band Histoire d'A, were the last to perform. They came off stage at 1 a.m. and the DJs picked it up from there.

It was then that Morgane began, in the words of Nicolas and Mathieu, to make a spectacle of herself.

Lap-dancing, provocative poses . . .

Nicolas and Mathieu said they had tried to reason with her. She had drunk a few beers, but not that much. This was confirmed by the autopsy results, which revealed there was less than 0.9 grams of alcohol in her blood. Enough to release Morgane's inhibitions.

Nicolas Gravé and Clara Barthélémy then revealed another piece of information: they had been secretly dating for several weeks. The outing had been a pretext, and the three other passengers alibis. From 2 a.m. onwards Nic and Clara were kissing and cuddling on a Sea View sofa. They were oblivious to Morgane's disappearance until 6 a.m., when a guy ran in screaming, 'There's a dead body on the beach! Oh my God, there's a dead body on the beach!'

Mathieu and Océane had played gooseberry for a while, but by 3 a.m. they were bored with the dance floor. For the next hour they alternated between trying to make conversation over the loud music and dozing off on the sofas. They weren't paying much attention to what Morgane was up to. The last time they recalled seeing her was at 3.30 a.m., on the dance floor. Mathieu Picard said he wasn't worried when she disappeared because he'd assumed she would not be ending the evening alone. After the festival, the casino and beach had turned into one giant shag pad. He admitted that he'd half-heartedly tried his luck with Océane, but got nowhere even though she had drunk more than usual. The two of them had been friends since kindergarten, but unlike Morgane she wasn't one for flirting. In his words, she was a ball-breaker, just like her mother.

This left Captain Grima with a two-hour 'black hole' between the last sighting of Morgane and the discovery of her body at 5.30 a.m.

Or, to be precise, just under two hours. The Sea View cloakroom attendant, Sonia Thurau, a little blonde who resembled a trash goth Barbie doll, remembered seeing Morgane going out for a cigarette at about 3.40. She insisted there was no way she could have been mistaken; Morgane was the hottest customer in the place that night. Sonia described her as having sweat trickling down her face, her tight dress clinging to her thighs and see-through with perspiration, revealing fuchsia underwear.

'She was wearing her panties and her bra at that point,' Sonia confirmed.

'You're very observant,' Grima complimented her.

'Too right. I'd happily have eaten that little pussy of hers!'

Sonia Thurau's reply left the captain disconcerted, for her observant eye was at that moment savouring his own anatomy in a way that made it clear her sexual preferences were not exclusive. The next time they called Sonia in, he made sure she was interviewed by an officer who was nearing retirement age.

'Stepped outside for a cigarette . . .'

The captain thought about that detail for a long time after the interview.

Morgane Avril didn't smoke.

Another dead end.

While he continued his efforts to find more witnesses and reconstruct every minute of Morgane's evening, Captain Grima shifted his focus to the murder weapon.

The Burberry scarf.

On 19 July 2004, Judge Nadeau-Loquet sent him a message congratulating him on the significant progress in the investigation that had resulted from Grima pursuing an angle everyone else had overlooked.

A scarf. A scrap of fabric worth more than four hundred euros.

Grima took the time to check all the witness statements, to

72

cross-reference the different versions of events and eliminate pieces of information that seemed too far-fetched.

In the end, only three credible witnesses remembered the Burberry scarf.

Sonia Thurau, behind her cloakroom counter, pulled a face when the grizzled policeman showed up. But his questions jogged her memory of a customer she described as a 'daddy's boy'. Asked for more details, 'suntanned' was the only adjective she would agree to put in her statement. She rejected 'swarthy', 'Maghrebi', 'mixed race', and every other term the old cop suggested, insisting that the disco ball had made it impossible for her to tell the colour of his skin.

The suntanned daddy's boy had stopped by the cloakroom to check in his linen jacket and cashmere scarf. Not too many festival-goers wore that sort of gear, which was why Sonia remembered him.

'Was it a red scarf? A Burberry?'

She hadn't noticed the brand but, yes, it could easily have been a Burberry. Sonia hadn't seen the guy leave, so a colleague must have served him when he returned for his clothes, but none of them remembered.

Captain Grima considered the possibility that Sonia Thurau had invented this mysterious customer after reading newspaper accounts referring to 'the red-scarf killer'. But she seemed a reliable witness; when she wasn't running the casino cloakroom, Sonia was studying comparative European law. What's more, two other witnesses reported seeing a man with a scarf.

Mickey, a temporary bouncer who had spent the night of 5–6 June patrolling the car park where the sound of guitar riffs struggled to compete with the noise of the waves, recalled seeing a man smoking under the cliff, near the casino bins, who seemed to be wearing a jacket and a scarf. He hadn't been able to make out the colour. Neither could he remember the time. After three in the morning, that was all he could be sure of, because he had taken a break. He couldn't be more precise than that. He was alone, Mickey was sure of it.

'Did you get the impression he was waiting for somebody?' Grima asked.

'Possibly.'

'A girl?'

'Could be . . . or some mates. I carried on making my rounds.'

That was all Mickey had seen: a silhouette glimpsed between the halo of a street lamp and the beam of his torch. But it was around the time that Morgane Avril was seen leaving the Sea View . . . And that was the last time she was seen alive.

The third witness, Vincent Carré, a twenty-one-year-old chemistry student, had arrived at Bréauté, the nearest station to Yport, at around 5 p.m. Coaches had been laid on to transport festival-goers to the concert, so Vincent joined the line of people waiting to board. He found himself standing beside a guy who seemed to be about the same age as him, but unlike everyone else there he was elegantly dressed: white shirt, polished pumps, jacket over his shoulder and red scarf around his neck.

'What's with the fancy get-up?' Vincent had asked.

'Girls like it.'

'Are you here for the music or the girls?'

Vincent Carré clearly remembered his reply.

'The music or the girls? Are you serious? Good music is rare, and you're not going to find the next Hendrix playing Yport! But the girls . . . Hey, girls are beautiful everywhere!'

When the coach arrived, Vincent hadn't taken the seat next to the guy in the scarf. Not really his tribe. They had both plugged in their headphones. End of story.

Except Vincent had seen the guy with the scarf again at the Sea View. He was dancing in the crowd, and most of the time he was hanging around the most beautiful girl in the place, Morgane, though Vincent didn't know her name at the point. It was obvious the guy was trying to chat her up.

He wasn't wearing his scarf on the dance floor, but dozens of other witnesses confirmed that there was a guy prowling around Morgane. Océane and Mathieu had seen him too. Everybody, Vincent included, contributed to the photofit. It showed a rather square, handsome face, brown eyes, very brown complexion, perhaps even, although they couldn't be certain, of North African origin. A composite artist worked for two days putting together a sketch that was as vague as it was banal. But it was distributed everywhere. Hundreds of responses, all checked, led nowhere. Not that Captain Grima had entertained any real hope in the portrait of a man glimpsed in the semi-darkness of a disco, when witnesses had had no idea of the tragedy that would unfold, no reason to etch that face in their memory.

Vincent Carré spotted the stranger again the following morning. By that time Yport was in turmoil: Morgane Avril's corpse had just been discovered and the police were patrolling the village. The guy was standing in the Place Jean-Paul Laurens, outside the bakery, with his jacket draped over his shoulder. Vincent passed in front of him, almost running; after falling into bed, exhausted, at 2 a.m., he'd woken this morning to the news that a girl had been found dead on the beach! Raped! Like every other male in the vicinity, he'd been told to report to the police so they could collect a DNA sample . . . When he passed in front of the stranger, Vincent Carré had no idea who had been killed, or how.

The guy had waved a hand in greeting. If he hadn't, Vincent would have passed him without noticing. When they spoke, there was no mention of the dead girl. Vincent Carré couldn't say why. He had the impression that the stranger wasn't aware that there'd been a murder. Either that or he didn't give a shit.

'So, did you enjoy the concert?' Vincent had asked.

The other man had burst out laughing. 'Come on . . .'

'And the local girls?'

'Pretty. Very pretty.'

'So I saw – you didn't go for the ugliest one.'

'No, only the hottest would do . . .'

Vincent Carré had put him down as a poser. He'd also noticed that the stranger was no longer wearing his red scarf.

'Did you lose your scarf?'

'I gave it to the girl,' the stranger said. 'As a souvenir.'

'Will you be seeing her again?'

75

'I very much doubt it.'

He had given a laugh that the psychologists would ask Vincent to describe again and again, asking him to elaborate on the finer nuances.

Did it seem spontaneous? Forced? Cynical? Sadistic?

Vincent had no idea. The one thing that stuck in his mind was the stranger's answer to his final question.

'Are you taking the bus?' Vincent had asked.

'No, I'm off to see my folks. They have a second home on the Normandy coast.'

The crux of the Morgane Avril case.

Naturally the police did all they could to verify the credibility of Vincent Carré's testimony. He seemed reliable, though the police were concerned about the gap in his schedule. Vincent had gone to bed at about two in the morning, leaving his mates to carry on partying without him. That wasn't like him . . .

When Captain Grima questioned him about it, Vincent said that he'd been tired, that he'd had a hard week. When pressed, he became indignant. How dare the police treat him like a suspect when his testimony had provided them with a breakthrough in the case. He had a point; Grima had no reason to suspect Vincent Carré any more than any other customer at the Sea View. Besides, his DNA didn't match the rapist's.

So they were looking for a boy of about twenty whose parents owned a second home on the Normandy coast. Captain Grima discovered at this point that there were over thirty-five thousand second homes in the region. Finding the right one proved impossible, despite teams of officers going door-to-door for weeks, photofit in hand, in ever-increasing circles, starting with the closest, Étretat, then Saint-Valéry-en-Caux, then Honfleur, then Deauville, Cabourg, Dieppe . . .

All in vain.

The stranger in the red scarf had vanished without trace.

Captain Grima delivered his report to Judge Nadeau-Loquet on

20 August 2004. By that time the investigation had been stalled for almost five weeks. No new evidence, but Grima remained convinced that Morgane Avril had agreed to follow the stranger who'd been seen with her on the dance floor. He had retrieved his jacket and his Burberry scarf from the cloakroom without anyone noticing, and then he had waited in the car park for Morgane. They had probably gone for a swim together in some secluded spot. Then things turned nasty.

Morgane has gone as far as she's willing to, but the stranger refuses to take no for an answer. He rapes her, panics, strangles her, carries her corpse to the top of the cliff and throws her off, perhaps to make it look like a suicide.

Then he disappears . . .

Despite his failure to apprehend the suspect, Captain Grima concluded his report to Judge Nadeau-Loquet on an optimistic note. Morgane Avril's murderer had been partially identified. Eventually, he would lower his guard and someone would spot him, either on the Normandy coast or elsewhere. But there was one thing Captain Grima was certain of:

Morgane Avril's killer would never strike again.

This was a young man from a well-to-do family, cultured, well-educated, who had made the biggest mistake of his life that night in Yport. He would live with that monstrous secret buried deep inside him. Until his death.

If they didn't catch him before then . . .

The police report unleashed the fury of the Avril clan.

Carmen Avril and her family, through their lawyer, took issue with Captain Grima's theory. As far as they were concerned, the murderer was a pervert, a predator whose actions were premeditated. They pointed to Vincent Carré's account of the stranger with the red scarf on the morning after the murder, waiting calmly for his parents to come and get him, untroubled by the police manhunt for Morgane's killer.

Police, lawyers and judges spent hours discussing the brief exchange reported by Vincent Carré:

'Did you lose your scarf?'

'I gave it to the girl. As a souvenir.'

'Will you be seeing her again?'

'I very much doubt it.'

Did these sound like the words of a young man who had slipped up and committed a murder that he would regret for the rest of his days? Or the gloating of a cynical and cold-blooded criminal? Or were they the words of an innocent man – albeit one who had failed to present himself to the police so that he could be eliminated?

On 23 August, *Le Havre Libre* quoted Captain Grima's dismissive response to the suggestion that Morgane's murder had been premeditated. He found it unbelievable that the killer could have devised a plan that would allow him to approach and then attack Morgane Avril without being seen. And why the dip in the sea? Why the Burberry scarf?

Then, on 26 August 2004, his theory was blown to pieces.

Along with his credibility.

All that effort he'd put in, the sleepless nights away from home, missing three months of his baby daughter's life in the process – wasted.

Overnight, the case of the red Burberry scarf turned into a drama of such magnitude it surpassed anything Captain Grima could have imagined.

The sound of the bell dragged me from my reading.

It rang out continuously, as if summoning a ship's crew to assemble on deck.

André's voice boomed in the corridor:

'Jamal! Dinner time!'

I looked at the clock on my bedside table: 7.17 p.m.

Shit!

11

Will you be seeing her again?

I made my way down the steps into the dining room, which was big enough to accommodate over thirty people, with most of the tables commanding a view of the sea. In February, however, the Sirène felt more like a family boarding house than a hotel restaurant. Tonight, only a handful of the tables were occupied. There were two pensioners, stopping for one night on their way to Mont St Michel. An English couple who had arrived on the ferry to Dieppe with their red-faced baby. A man in a tie, sitting alone, like a lost sales rep.

And a surprise guest, who greeted me with the words:

'You're late, Jamal.'

Mona!

She was dining alone at her table, sitting over her plate of whelks armed with a small stainless-steel skewer. The pensioners ate in silence a few tables away. In the other corner of the room, the English couple were struggling to make their baby eat vegetables.

Mona indicated the chair in front of her. 'Would you rather eat on your own, or will you join me?'

How could I refuse?

As soon as I sat down, André appeared with my plate and my cutlery. He vanished with a complicit smile; I couldn't tell whether it was meant for her or for me.

'You sneaky little thing! Did you arrive at the Sirène this morning?' That explained her mysterious comment at the police station, about seeing me later. Her eyes sparkled with delight at having duped me.

'That's right. Yesterday, I was prospecting on Veules-les-Roses, but now I have to move on to the pebble beaches between the oil terminal at Antifer and the nuclear plant at Paluel. When you came back from your jog this morning I was standing right behind you, at the counter, but you didn't notice me.'

Hardly surprising, given that was the moment André handed me the first envelope.

'And did you manage to persuade the police to approve your permit?'

'Yes! But I had to sleep with half the station. What about you, no new suicides?'

'Not to my knowledge.'

André arrived with my whelks and mayonnaise at that moment. He must have heard the 'no new suicides' remark, but showed no sign of it.

'Let's have a bottle of wine,' Mona suggested. 'I'll get this!'

I protested for form's sake, but Mona insisted.

'I'll put it on expenses. My company's not short of a euro or two. P@nshee Computer Technologies must have made almost five billion in profits last year. There's no reason why Key Biscayne retirees should be the only ones to profit from that, is there?'

She ordered a 2009 white Burgundy, a Vougeot Chardonnay premier cru.

Seventy-five euros! My entire budget for the week.

A long silence set in between us. I had no desire to talk about that morning's suicide, about the Burberry scarf, even less about the Morgane Avril case. Mona seemed to offer a pleasant interlude amid this torrent of unanswered questions and impossible coincidences.

My gaze darted about the room, from the romantic paintings of storms over the cliff, to the sailors' knots displayed in wood and copper frames, the 'Welcome aboard' lifebelt, the giant compass hanging from the beam. I lingered on these maritime knick-knacks, knowing that the alternative would be to risk drowning in Mona's cleavage.

She had undone another button on her blouse since I saw her that afternoon.

To seduce me, or to persuade the police to stamp her permit?

Mona was the first to break the silence.

'Do you know how the CEO of P@nshee made his fortune?'

'No idea . . .'

'It's an incredible story. You'll love this, Jamal. Panshee Kumar Shinde is his name, he arrived in San Francisco in the mid-seventies as a poor Indian immigrant without a rupee to his name. By night he cleaned toilets in downtown offices, and by day he took classes in management at one of those colleges that rips off foreign students by charging them thousands of dollars, leaving them in debt for three generations. Halfway through the course, Panshee was assigned a business creation project. He had to draw up a marketing plan, an amortisation programme – the whole shebang. Exhausted by the work he did at night, he hadn't managed to write a single line. The night before he was due to hand in his work, he was cleaning the toilets of the Transamerica Pyramid, forty-seventh floor, with no idea what business he could create, even a virtual one. More prosaically, he was raging against the idiots who clogged the toilets with tissues or sheets of A4 when there was no toilet paper . . .'

Mona took a sip of Chardonnay before going on:

'And then he had the idea—'

'In the toilets?'

'Yes – the most idiotic idea in the universe. Rather than putting a standard twenty-metre roll of toilet paper in offices, the same as the ones you'd use at home, why not install a much longer roll? Two hundred, three hundred metres, locked up in a metal dispenser. He started with that, for lack of anything better, and spent the rest of the night drafting his project. The next day, he was about to get off the subway train to go to his class when at the last moment he changed his mind. He stayed on the train, got off five stops later, at West Portal, and went into the Wells Fargo office to sell his project and apply for the patent.'

'Did it work?'

'Before the year was out he was a multi-billionaire. One of the hundred richest people in the world. Do you know a single public building that doesn't have one of those toilet-paper dispensers? Can you imagine how many metres of toilet paper are rolled out every day from those things?'

Mona finished her glass and continued:

'It was the most lucrative patent of the century! Panshee went on to invest in computer technology, then he bought an island in Micronesia. They say he never wears clothes and wipes his bum with palm fronds.'

'Is that true?'

She burst out laughing. 'What do you think?'

I hesitated for a moment.

'You made it all up?'

'Perhaps. I love telling stories.'

I wanted to applaud, to hold her in my arms, run outside with her to the sea wall and laugh all night beneath the moon. I had never met a girl I had so much in common with. That offbeat sense of humour, as if she's not quite living in the real world, caught somewhere between the cars rumbling in the street below and the stars up above. For the second time that day I thought about Djamila. Mona reminded me of my grandmother, the Sheherezade of Drancy. Every Saturday evening all the kids used to gather to listen to her stories, Géricault Tower, staircase C – until they bunged Djamila in a care home at Blanc-Mesnil and the nurses reduced her fabulous stories to incoherent rantings, proof of advanced Alzheimer's. I was eight years old. I have never forgotten any of her stories.

André took advantage of my preoccupation to remove my plate and set down a bowl of mussels. A brief hesitation on his part told me that he wanted to talk, probably about the suicide that he had just heard us discussing. The news had spread: a girl found dead after leaping off the cliff. Perhaps the fact that someone had tried to strangle her had got out as well . . .

I imagined the panic in the fishermen's houses.

Ten years later, had the Burberry-scarf rapist returned?

'What about you?' Mona suddenly asked me.

'Me?'

'Yes! Your turn to tell me an amazing story.'

I shook my head, all out of inspiration, as if sorting through the mussels had exhausted all my powers of invention. Mona stamped her foot.

'Don't disappoint me, Jamal! I wouldn't have invited you to my table if I hadn't been sure that you were going to surprise me. Come on, something crazy!'

I took a moment to wipe my fingers on my napkin. Three tables away, the pensioners were too engrossed in their smartphones to pay any attention to each other.

'OK, Mona. You've asked for it. A crazy thing? Here you go: I've found a revolutionary way of getting off with girls. A sure-fire method of luring the most beautiful ones into bed.'

I had Mona's attention. She sat up straight, opened her eyes wide and parted her lips.

'You don't believe me?' I asked.

'I'm waiting for you to show me some proof.'

I took out my wallet and removed a small business card. I placed it on the table, concealing it with my palm so that Mona couldn't read it.

'There's my secret weapon.'

'Ah,' Mona said, exaggerating her disappointment.

I pushed the card towards her without revealing it.

'For ten years I've never gone out without my cards. I always have a few in my pocket. As I go about my day, commuting to work, walking the city streets, every now and then I happen upon a girl I like. Without stopping, without giving her the chance to get a proper look at me, I slip one of these cards into her hand.'

I opened my hand and read the card.

Dear Mademoiselle,

I have calculated that every day I see several thousand women in the streets of Paris. Every day I give a card to one of those women, sometimes two, rarely three, never more.

One woman out of several thousand.

You. Today.

You are different. In this crowd, something sets you apart from all the others.

If there is a man who loves you and you are happy with him, I hope you will still be touched by my gesture.

If you aren't loved, that's an injustice. Because you deserve to be. More than anyone else.

In my eyes.

Thank you for this magic moment.

jamalsalaoui@yahoo.fr

I gave the card to Mona and she snatched it up as if it were a treasure map.

'Whoa! And this works?'

I emptied my glass, savouring it. One euro per centilitre.

'It's infallible! At worst, the woman feels flattered. At best, she falls for it. I play on the element of surprise, on their ego, on the contrast between Parisian indifference and my little touch of romanticism. You see, Mona, it's the ideal compromise between virtual flirting on hook-up sites and the clumsy passes that girls constantly have to put up with in the street.'

Mona reached for the bottle and topped up our glasses. She whistled between her teeth.

'One girl in thousands. How do you choose?'

'I'm not sure how to explain it. If there's one thing I've never understood it's love at first sight. Frankly, Mona, almost all women are charming, almost all of them have a little something that would make you fall in love with them, to love them for a lifetime without regret. But when it comes to love at first sight, that isn't enough . . . At least one woman in three is really pretty if she wants to be. And at least one woman in ten – in twenty, perhaps, is perfect. Each in her own unique way, but perfect. But love at first sight comes from a look that blows me away. Women who can leave me thunderstruck like that – I come across one of those per metro carriage, ten outside every café in a Paris square in the sun, a hundred on a summer beach . . .'

Mona stopped devouring mussels and studied me intently.

'You're not an easy one to work out, Jamal. Are you the worst kind of sexist, or the inventor of post-romanticism?'

She paused, as if looking for the flaw in my method.

'And you really only hand out three cards a day?'

I mimed the expression of a sheepish child who's just been caught out.

'Are you kidding? Some days I hand out several hundred!'

She burst out laughing. 'You fraud! And do they respond?'

'Seriously?'

'Yes.'

'I have a response rate of almost eighty per cent . . . Almost everyone succumbs after three emails. I've slept with the most beautiful girls in the capital. I have a better strike rate than the boss of the biggest modelling agency in Paris.'

'Are you having me on?'

'Maybe, I like making up stories.'

Mona raises her glass of Chardonnay and clinks it against mine.

'Lovely, Jamal. Nil-all draw.'

After a moment's hesitation, she asked: 'If you'd bumped into me in the street, would you have given me a card?'

I knew that I mustn't answer too quickly. I drank in every detail: her skin, the blusher on her cheekbones, the shadows of her eyelashes on her beautiful turned-up nose. Mona played along, assuming a pose and staring at the sea so that I could admire her profile. Then she stretched, offering me her breasts and her throat.

At last I replied, weighing each syllable:

'Yes, and I would only have handed out one card that day.'

Mona blushed. For the first time, I sensed she was embarrassed.

'Liar!' she managed to say.

Then she took a long breath before asking her next question.

'And your . . . your leg . . . Was it an accident?'

In the end, she was no different to the others. She couldn't resist asking. I had my answer ready. I'd had it ready for years.

'Yes. Porte Maillot. The most beautiful girl was waiting on the other side of the carriage, I couldn't let her go without giving her a card . . . I jumped on to the tracks, but the train arrived at that very moment!'

She laughed.

'Idiot! Will you tell me one day?'

'I promise.'

'You're a funny guy, Jamal. Funny, but a liar! Besides, I'm sure that you wouldn't have given me your card. I reckon you go for romantic women, femmes fatales. Not direct girls like me. If you ask me, that's the problem with your technique: you collect women like Panini stickers, but you don't get the ones you need!'

'Thanks for the advice.'

'Excuse me,' said a voice behind us.

André was standing there, holding two bowls of îles flottantes. He set them down, narrowly avoiding a tsunami, then blurted out the question that had been bothering him.

'Jamal, just now you were talking about a suicide. Is that . . . is that recent?'

Clearly, André knew nothing about this morning's accident. Strange!

I set out the facts, neglecting to mention that I had found the Burberry scarf stuck to a piece of barbed wire on the cliff, and that it had been inexplicably found around Magali Verron's neck. The further I got into my story, the wider André's eyes grew. When I paused, the proprietor of the Sirène, white as his napkins, stammered.

'Your story reminds me—'

I interrupted him.

'The rape of Morgane Avril. Ten years ago.'

André slowly nodded.

'I was there,' he went on. 'You might say I had a front-row seat! The Avril girl died right in front of my window. The Riff on the Cliff festival was a godsend for me. I must have sold litres of mussels, chips and kebabs, my tables filled the whole of the sea wall, the weather was good that evening, young people came from all over the place. It was the first and last time such an event was held in Yport.'

'I understand.' I couldn't find anything better to say.

'I'm not going to complain,' André said. 'After the murder my hotel was full for six months. Journalists, police, forensic experts, witnesses, lawyers.'

'So that's good news, then,' Mona said. 'With this new death, your hotel will be full again!'

I wasn't sure that André would enjoy Mona's sense of humour as much as I did. He remained silent for a long time.

'I only hope,' he added at last, 'that there won't be any more.'

'More what?'

'More victims.'

'One every ten years,' Mona carried on. 'That gives you a bit of a margin.'

André gave her a strange look, which passed through Mona as if she didn't exist. I had the feeling it wasn't so much contempt for Mona's misplaced humour as the hope that we would share his concern. I turned towards him.

'Why, André? Why would there be more victims?'

He looked as if he had aged ten years in a single evening. He pulled up a chair and sat down beside us. He studied the black horizon for a long time, then spoke in a low voice.

'So you don't know the whole story, Jamal? You only know about Morgane Avril?'

I thought again of the first lines of the newspaper articles I had read before dinner, the collapse of Captain Grima's theory, the case assuming a national dimension.

'Four months after the murder of Morgane Avril,' André went on, 'there was a second crime. A girl from Elbeuf, near Rouen. It happened in Basse-Normandie, another seaside town, towards the end of the holidays. She was in charge of a camp for teenagers. The same rapist. The same sperm. Strangled with a red Burberry scarf. Panic broke out in Normandy after that! They were afraid that the serial killer would keep going . . . But it stopped there . . . Two girls . . .'

He paused for a long time.

'Until this morning.'

I tried to suggest a rational explanation: 'So the sick bastard must have been in jail for ten years, then he got out and started all over again?'

'He was never caught,' André said mournfully.

He remained thoughtful, lost in his memories. The chemical-tasting îles flottantes melted gently into their sea of cream. At last André went off to clear the table of the English couple, who had disappeared with their child, leaving behind them a sea of green purée.

Mona contemplated her dessert as if it were an ice floe that had fallen victim to global warming.

'Terrible business.'

I thought for a while without even looking up at her.

Two murders.

A rapist who had gone into hiding for ten years and then struck again this morning.

Except that this time he hadn't killed his victim.

Magali had thrown herself from the top of the cliff. After twisting the scarf around her neck.

The scarf covered with my prints.

Someone knew. Someone was playing with me, and was going to drip-feed me information.

Why me? What did I have to do with this whole business?

Mona's fingers played with my card.

'Shall we go?' she said.

I didn't reply. She seemed disappointed by the turn that the end of the meal had taken, as if she had been plunged too brutally into reality. She read out loud some of the words from my card.

'"Thank you for this magic moment." Let me tell you something, Jamal. I would have loved for a stranger to slip a note like that into my hand on a suburban station platform. I think I'd have allowed myself to be seduced, whatever happened.'

She took the time to look out of the bay window, into the light from the street lamps, the dance of the moored fishing boats. Empty. Or crewed by ghosts. Then she added:

'But having dinner with a panoramic view of the sea isn't bad either.'

She pushed back her chair and got to her feet. I rubbed my eyes, troubled by the unlikely series of events that had occurred since this morning, then I gave her a smile. Mona seemed to like it.

'I have a rule, Jamal. When I like a guy, I always sleep with him on the first date.'

12

Why me?

Mona opened the window. The sound of pebbles rolled by the waves invaded the room, making it feel like the cabin of a boat on the open sea. Mona was standing between the two curtains, naked, offering her skin to the flecks of foam carried by the wind as the waves crashed against the sea wall.

I was lying on the bed, admiring the view. The swell of Mona's hips, her round bottom, her legs – the legs of a mermaid who had bade farewell to the ocean. The moon painted the night in chiaroscuro. The lights on the deserted beach danced on Mona; the neon red of the casino, the sandy yellow of the halogen lamps.

She turned. A pair of brown hazelnuts stood out on the golden dunes of her breasts. A few stray red tendrils grew from her shaved pubes.

Splendid.

In bed, once she had untied the elastic that held her ponytail, Mona's hair had cascaded to her shoulders, lending unfamiliar volume to her mousy face. A gravity, almost – until she dispelled it with an explosion of laughter.

With Mona, everything was a game. A game filled with energy and invention, like the games of childhood. Hide-and-seek. Tag. Close your eyes, give me your hand, open your lips.

I had never experienced anything like it.

Neither of us had a contraceptive – she didn't care. She pressed gently on my lower back to make me stay inside her.

She whispered my name before she came.

I looked at the alarm clock. Ten past three in the morning.

Mona pushed the window ajar and came towards me. I imagined her picking up one of the seashells stuck to the frame of the wall and covering her sex with it, like Botticelli's Venus.

'I have a pied-à-terre in Vaucottes,' she said. 'Do you know it?'

I knew it. I passed Vaucottes every morning on my run. That wooded valley with its little patch of beach was one of the prettiest oases along the entire coast. The only dwellings were a handful of nineteenth-century baroque villas.

'My thesis supervisor has a house there,' Mona said. 'He gave me the keys, but I haven't set foot in the place yet. Judging by the photographs, it's an old cabin, elegant and sinister, like something out of *Psycho* . . .'

'Did you sleep with him?'

She seemed almost surprised by the question.

'Don't be ridiculous! I'm as boring at work as I'm fun at sex. If I were to start combining the two . . . Disaster!'

She jumped on to the bed and began trailing her fingers along my back.

'Tired already? Do you go running very early? My mother always warned me: "Darling, never sleep with an elite athlete!"'

I kissed her on the lips and placed my hand on her right breast.

'Give me a few minutes. OK?'

I didn't wait for her reply. I slipped on a pair of underpants and turned on my laptop, on the desk facing the bed. As I'd expected, this prompted a barrage of sarcastic remarks from Mona.

'I've pulled a geek! What are you doing? Tweeting to tell the world that you've just lost your virginity to the hottest girl on the coast?'

I sketched a smile. 'No, it's what André was telling us earlier. That double rape . . .'

'The one a decade ago, or yours, from this morning?'

'The one from ten years ago.'

'Can't it wait?'

No. I need to know.

'Give me two seconds, Mona. Then I'll tell you the craziest thing you've ever heard.'

I'd decided to tell Mona everything, from the first time I caught sight of the Burberry scarf on the barbed wire to the last time I saw it: wrapped round the neck of the beautiful young suicide.

My old laptop took ages to get going.

'You couldn't do me a favour, Mona? In my jacket pocket, in my wallet, there's the password for the Wi-Fi here.'

The sheet slid slowly over Mona's curves as she wriggled across the bed to pick up my things. She called out the series of numbers and letters.

I typed in a few initial words at random.

Serial killer
Lower Normandy
2004
Burberry scarf

Google offered me a hundred answers, all along the same lines. Some words came up again and again in the headlines or summaries of the articles.

Myrtille Camus
Thursday 26 August 2004
Isigny-sur-Mer Leisure Centre
Raped
Murdered

One of the names settled in my head.

Isigny-sur-Mer

Though I couldn't think why. I wasn't even able to locate the village on the Normandy coast. I tried to concentrate, but at that moment Mona's voice rang out behind my back.

'I see through your disguise – you're an undercover cop!'

A cop?

Mona had gone insane! Startled, I turned to face her.

'Why would you say that?'

She waved a dented gold sheriff's star under my nose.

My star!

Mona hadn't merely looked for my wallet, she had searched all the pockets of my jacket.

'A childhood souvenir?' Mona asked.

'Exactly. Put it back, please.'

I thought again of that autumn morning when the social worker had delivered me home to my mother's. I was seven years old. Instead of telling me off, my mother had taken me to the toy shop in the shopping centre on the other side of the dual carriageway. At the time I was watching a lot of videos of old westerns that my uncle Kamel collected. My mother had bought me that sheriff's star that couldn't have been worth more than five francs and fixed it to my jacket, then brought me home and plonked me down in front of a cowboy film. She wanted me to understand what side of the law I was to put myself on. For ever.

'Did you write those words?'

Instead of putting my star away, Mona was examining it from every angle.

'Five verbs,' she went on. 'One on each point.'

Become

Make

Have

Be

Pay

I sighed.

'They're principles, Mona. Guidelines, if you prefer. It's a kind of compass.'

'Tell me!'

Mona's eyes gleamed. It was too late to tear that star from her hands. The sheet had slipped once and for all from her bottom, but I felt even more naked than her. Feigning indifference, I plunged back into the Google answers.

'Seriously,' Mona pressed. 'What's with these five verbs?'

'My compass. I told you.'

Again I pretended to be focused on my computer screen while she carried on rummaging in my wallet. A few seconds later she triumphantly displayed a piece of paper folded into four.

'Found it!' she shouted.

No one had ever gone through my belongings like that, no one had ever known about the five lines written on that piece of paper, but I did nothing to stop her from reading them.

As she read them out loud, I thought I could feel her heart beating beneath her breast.

1. *Become* – the first disabled athlete to run the Mont Blanc Ultra-Trail.
2. *Make* – love to a woman more beautiful than me.
3. *Have* – a child.
4. *Be* – mourned by a woman when I die.
5. *Pay* – my debt before I die.

She fell silent and looked at me for a long time.

'I don't understand, Jamal. Can you explain it for me?'

I clicked on another article.

'Can you explain it for me?' Mona said again.

Reluctantly, I took my eyes off the screen.

'I'm sure you've worked it out already, Mona. They're what you might call my guiding principles. Ambitions, if you like. The goals I set myself to get over my disability. If possible, I want to tick those five boxes before I die. I don't care when my ashes are scattered, as long as I've achieved those five goals.'

'You're crazy!'

'Isn't that what attracted you to me?'

I clicked on a PDF.

France-Soir
The serial killer terrifying Normandy. Witnesses give a vague description of a man in his twenties wearing a blue and white Adidas cap.

'Goal number one,' Mona observed. 'The Mont Blanc run. I get that one. You're training for it every morning. It's at the end of the summer, isn't it? You've got plenty of time. Goal number one achieved, then!'

I smiled in spite of myself. Did she have any idea of the difficulty of the course and the magnitude of the feat that I had taken it into my head to accomplish? The biggest trail in the world? My child-hood dream. Not to mention the qualifying runs in the months leading up to the event . . .

'OK,' she went on sarcastically. 'Thanks to me, you can also tick box number two: *Make love to a woman more beautiful than me!*'

Mona threw off the covers with a flick of her heel and stretched out her naked body on the bed as if inviting my approval.

What could I say? She was, by some way, the most beautiful girl I'd ever slept with.

Instead of waiting for a reply, Mona went on:

'Goals three and four. A child. A grieving widow. OK, Jamal, but there's an important detail missing here. Are you supposed to achieve all these goals with the same woman? The woman in number two?'

I carried on staring at the screen.

'So?' Mona went on. 'Lover, mother and widow. One, two or three women?'

'It doesn't matter.'

'Liar!'

'No – the woman mourning as she scatters my ashes could be my daughter when I'm very old.'

'Good point! Let's finish with goal number five: *pay my debt before I die*. Is that like a debt to society? What did you do? Kill someone?'

I sat on the bed and rested my hand on her hip.

'It refers to the debt we all have: to pay for our own life by saving another, to be useful.'

'You haven't done too well on that score! You couldn't even stop little Magali from jumping off the cliff!'

My hand slid along her curves. It seemed nothing was taboo where Mona was concerned. I had never talked to anybody about the five directions on my compass, not even Ibou or Ophélie. I tried to explain it to her:

'It could also refer to stopping a murderer. Preventing him from striking again.'

'The Burberry scarf rapist?'

'For example.'

Mona put one hand over my eyes and gently took my hand with the other, guiding it across her body.

'Forget him . . .'

The green LEDs of the alarm clock showed 4.03. We had made love again, then I had stayed there, wrapped between Mona's legs, and told her all about the mystery of the red scarf around Magali Verron's neck. I finished with a question.

'Do you think I should tell the police what I've just told you?'

'I don't know. I mean, there's nothing odd about you finding that Burberry scarf caught on the fence. The guy who raped Magali Verron must have panicked when he heard you coming, and left it where it was. But then . . .'

Mona frowned, deep in thought. Then she sat up.

'I know! The rapist must have been wearing a mask. Or a balaclava. Or maybe Magali didn't have time to study his face. When she saw you a few minutes later, holding the scarf, she thought her attacker had come back. She thought you were him!'

96

I ran through the scene in my head. I remembered the words that Magali had said before she jumped.

Don't come any closer.
If you take so much as a step, I'll jump . . .
Keep running. Go! Get out of here, now!

How could I have been so stupid? I had frightened her like a hunter cornering a rabbit. Paralysed with terror, she'd have done anything to avoid falling into the hands of the man who'd raped her. Even take her own life.

Mona's hypothesis chilled me.

If I hadn't approached with that scarf in my hand, Magali wouldn't have jumped.

Oblivious to my distress, Mona carried on pursuing her train of thought.

'Jamal, that might even explain why she wrapped that scarf around her neck as she fell . . .'

She paused for a second.

'To accuse you!'

To accuse me?

My naked skin suddenly seemed repulsive – how could Mona bear to touch it? I moved away. This time she noticed that I was upset and laid a hand my shoulder.

On the bedside table, the sheriff's star reflected the light of the ship's lamp. She began to caress me.

'Don't worry about it, Jamal. You're not responsible. You couldn't have known.'

I leapt to my feet. Mona's fingers were left clutching at thin air.

'You didn't do anything wrong, Jamal! You're innocent. You have nothing to fear from the police. Your sperm won't be a match for the sperm of Magali Verron's rapist, any more than it's a match for the man who raped those two girls ten years ago.'

I stared through the window at the black cliffs. Mona said again behind my back:

'You have nothing to fear from the police, Jamal.'
But she was wrong.
She was terribly wrong.
I would soon discover just how wrong she was.

13

Into the hands of her executioner?

At 10.22 the envelope was placed on the bench beside me. I was gazing out at the ten or so caiques – the local fishing boats – slumbering on the pebbles. Left high and dry by the outgoing tide. In the channel that had been dug in the foreshore to make it easier for boats to reach the sea, two windsurfers were setting up their wishbones. The younger of the two, his long blond mane bleached by the seawater, had painted a Viking helmet on his board; the other, a greying woman in her forties, had opted for a stylised version of the two leopards of Normandy in gold on a red background.

These were the real adventurers! Some sports you could only truly engage in by taking on the elements – the icy wind, the grey sea, the chalk cliffs. Those guys surfing beneath the palm trees of Honolulu or Sydney in their Bermuda shorts were lightweights in comparison.

I exchanged a conspiratorial smile with them. I wasn't ready to open the envelope yet. I wanted to savour the morning calm a while longer.

I had woken at about 7.30. The first thing I did was to reach for my sheriff's star and pin it to the blouse that Mona had thrown on the side of the bed. Right over her heart.

'Keep it, Mona,' I had murmured sleepily. 'You can have it.'

Her warm body was pressed against mine.

'Whoa! Big responsibility!'

'Huge!'

Then I had gone back to sleep. An hour later, Mona slipped away, leaving me a note.

Have to go to work. I'll be somewhere on the beach.

By the time I went down to the lobby of the Sirène in my running gear it was almost nine o'clock.

'I see the New Year resolutions have gone out the window,' André joked, consulting his watch. 'Lying in bed all morning isn't going to get you a place on the Ultra-Trail . . .'

'Extenuating circumstances, don't you think? She's a pretty girl . . .'

'What girl?' André said to me with a wink.

Given the average age of his customers, he couldn't have got many chances to play matchmaker.

I'd been planning on a fast and intense run, about fifteen kilometres due west, towards Étretat, before turning along the Ramendeuses path to the Valleuse de Grainval. I glanced at the weather forecast before setting off:

Risk of avalanche
Prolonged heavy snowfall
Gales expected late morning
-15 °C
05350 Saint-Véran
Hautes-Alpes

André's daily joke made me shiver in spite of myself. Outside, the beautiful light gave an illusion of warmth. I set off in a light breeze. By the time I reached the cliff path, the stiff grass crunched beneath my feet.

About halfway through my run I passed above Vaucottes. I was panting a little and wondered which of these strange goblin houses lost in a forest of ogres belonged to Mona's thesis supervisor. When I headed back towards Yport by the Sentier du Calvaire, I found myself face to face with the postman's van.

He looked at me as if I were a kid asking for the postcard from his girlfriend.

'An envelope? In the name of Jamal Salaoui? Yes, there was one today, but I've already dropped it off at the Sirène. You'll have to ask Dédé.'

I suspected as much, but I had another question for him.

'Is it possible to trace the sender of a parcel? By the franking, for example, if it's a company stamp rather than a postmark?'

The postman had the look of a teacher who was delighted to be given some overtime.

'Yes, in theory. But as regards your envelope, son, I happened to notice they'd used a franking machine. Any small business or government office in the region will have one just like it. If you're hoping to learn the identity of the secret admirer who's stalking you, you'll have to find another way.'

André was waiting for me by the front door of the Sirène, the envelope in his hands.

'Your subscription, Jamal! So what is it, *Storytime*, the *TV Guide* or *Playboy*?'

'*Gadgets Monthly*.'

I didn't want to open the envelope in my room. The sun was struggling to break through the clouds, so I headed for the bench on the sea wall. Even before I tore it open, I knew what the envelope contained.

The next instalment.

Everything I needed to follow the events of ten years ago.

By 10.29 the two windsurfers were gliding towards England. I reminded myself that I had less than four hours until my meeting with Piroz. It was time to open the envelope.

I took out the contents, gripping the pages with my fingers, stiff with cold, so the wind wouldn't scatter them.

Myrtille Camus case – Thursday, 26 August 2004

Victor Thouberville was up on his tractor, surveying his field. At first he thought some inconsiderate tourists had left their rubbish behind. Then he saw the torn dress. Followed by the girl's corpse.

Less than ten minutes later, two policemen from Isigny-sur-Mer arrived on the scene. They immediately made the connection with the Morgane Avril murder, three months earlier. Warning the two witnesses to the discovery, Victor Thouberville and his fifteen-year-old son, to be as discreet as possible, they got on to their superiors. A twenty-four-hour media embargo was imposed, long enough to confirm the link between the two crimes. After that, they couldn't hold back the news that would spread panic the length of the Normandy coastline.

Every headline featured the same two words: *Serial killer*.

Myrtille Camus was twenty years old. She worked as an activity leader at a camp for teenagers that had pitched its tents in Isigny-sur-Mer two weeks previously. The last witnesses to have seen her alive had passed her at about three o'clock on the Grandcamp trail. She was walking alone. It was her day off.

Every paragraph of the autopsy report confirmed investigators' worst fears.

Myrtille Camus had been raped, then strangled with a red cashmere scarf, probably a Burberry.

Preliminary DNA tests showed that Myrtille Camus's rapist was the same man who'd attacked Morgane Avril. Further testing confirmed the result beyond any possible doubt.

But the scarf and DNA results weren't the only indications that Morgane's killer had struck again.

Before being raped and strangled, Myrtille Camus had taken a dip in the sea. Naked – she didn't have a bathing costume with her and no trace of seawater was found on her underwear. No one had spotted her on any of the beaches along the route she'd taken. She had been wearing an elegant dress with big mauve hibiscus flowers on a sky-blue background. It was torn from top to bottom.

Like Morgane Avril, Myrtille Camus was still wearing her bra – mauve, to match the pattern on her dress – but her panties were missing. They were found the following day, in the channel of the Baie des Veys, stained with the rapist's sperm. The final similarity between the two cases was that Myrtille's bag had disappeared.

Investigators would spend months searching for it, without success.

The same heinous crime. The same rapist. The same murder weapon. The same level of violence.

The same modus operandi, including details that the police had never disclosed.

He's going to strike again.

After twenty-four hours, investigators were certain of one thing: *He won't stop there. The killer will strike again.*

An official statement was issued, thanking Captain Philippe Grima of Fécamp police station for his work over the last three months (there was no mention of his categorical assurance that Morgane Avril's murderer would never strike again), and announcing that responsibility for the investigation would henceforth be entrusted to a two-man team selected by the minister of the interior and the minister of justice.

Five years away from retirement, Commander Léo Bastinet of the Caen police department was renowned for his tact, organisational skills and British sense of humour. Bastinet was that rare creature, a leader admired both by his men and his superiors. He was teamed up with Paul-Hugo Lagarde, a young magistrate from Calvados, who'd quickly made a name for himself. Brilliant, ambitious and at ease with the media . . . but if he overstepped the mark, Bastinet would be the man to bring him back in line. The young judge was going to have to wait until the statute of limitations had run its course before publishing his bestselling account of the case.

The minister of the interior, alarmed by the spectre of a serial killer, had insisted on adding a third specialist to the team: criminal psychologist Ellen Nilsson. Thirty-six years old, with a long list of qualifications, she was given the task of monitoring the investigation and adding her insights as and when she saw fit.

The investigators' mission could be summed up in three commandments:

Work fast. Play things down. Catch this monster.

Given that the two victims had no ties, nothing whatsoever in common, they were dealing with a murderer who struck at random. Their task could not have been more difficullt.

More than five thousand people attended the funeral of Myrtille Camus in the church of Saint-Jean d'Elbeuf. Almost one in ten of the inhabitants of the town.

Myrtille Camus had become an icon. She deserved to be.

Everyone hated the murderer.

Everyone, perhaps, except her loved ones.

Charles and Louise Camus were well known in the town. Well known and well liked. Charles had been the curator of Elbeuf Museum for almost twenty years, and was regarded as an expert in everything from the archaeology of the Seine to nineteenth-century industrial machinery. Louise taught dance workshops and campaigned for the preservation of the town's famous circus-theatre.

A pair of humanists. Progressive. Moderate.

Louise and Charles had only one child, late in life. But for all that she was their greatest treasure, they resisted the urge to smother her in cotton wool.

Myrtille attended her mother's dance classes and the circus-theatre workshops. She also attended the local school in Le Puchot, perhaps an unusual choice given that its reputation was built on catering for children from deprived areas and those with special needs. At her birthday party in the Camus family home on the banks of the Seine, children from the richest families mingled with the daughters of the unemployed and the sons of African immigrants.

This was a deliberate choice by Louise and Charles. Not so much a political choice as a life choice. Myrtille was an only child, privileged and well loved. They wanted her to be beautiful not on the outside (which she was in any case, without their having to do anything about it) but on the inside. It was selfish and pretentious, when you think about it. They wanted her to embody their values – generosity, sharing, forgiveness – so that she could pass them on to the next generation of Camuses.

Even before Myrtille was born, Louise and Charles had been generous donors to the disadvantaged children of Elbeuf. In 1964, when the demise of the textile industry plunged half the local workforce into unemployment, they founded the Association of the Cloth of Gold. Every summer the Cloth of Gold ran camps for deprived youngsters who wouldn't otherwise have a holiday. Myrtille began attending the camps before she was old enough to walk; she was the mascot of the camp leaders who laid down the law in the dorms each summer (and on the pavements of the neighbourhood for the rest of the year).

In 1999 Louise and Charles handed over leadership of the organisation to Frédéric Saint-Michel, director of the community arts club and youth centre. He began training Myrtille as an activity leader as soon as she turned seventeen. Frédéric, who preferred to be called Chichin, like the lead guitarist of his favourite band, cultivated the appearance of a cool dude. He had long hair, a five o'clock shadow, and spoke in a low, serious voice. Thanks to his rigorous education and ten years as a scout, he projected a sense of morality that Charles and Louise found reassuring. Courtesy of a solo round-the-world trip in his late teens, he also possessed an air of madness that girls found charming, including some who were much younger than he was.

Including Myrtille.

In spite of the age difference, it seemed inevitable that Myrtille and Frédéric would fall in love. She was eighteen at the time and he was thirty-seven, but Louise and Charles raised no objection.

Frédéric was a lovely person.

Their wedding was scheduled for 2 October 2004. Myrtille's corpse still wore her engagement ring.

There would have been lots of people at Myrtille's wedding.

But perhaps not as many as attended her funeral.

The trio of investigators – the judge, the policeman and the psychological profiler – set to work immediately.

At first, Judge Lagarde's only task was to approve decisions made by the detective, while the criminal psychologist busied herself yawning over endless lists of DNA results. Since the murder of Morgane Avril, thousands of locals, summer visitors, campers from the Baie des Veys had contributed their DNA to the database.

With no result, except to eliminate them as suspects.

The photofit commissioned by Captain Grima – the one of the young man with the red Burberry scarf seen at Yport, the young man whose parents were believed to own a second home on the Normandy coast – had been distributed and displayed far and wide.

For want of any other alternative, he remained the number one suspect.

A ghost suspect.

No one in the area could remember having seen him. Either that or the portrait was a poor likeness.

Carmen Avril put pressure on the investigators. In September, *Femme Actuelle* magazine ran an interview with Morgane's mother. A quote from it was emblazoned across the cover:

If they'd listened to me, Myrtille Camus would still be alive!

Carmen Avril told the journalist she had known from the start that her daughter had fallen victim to a sadistic killer who had chosen her at random. Just as he had chosen Myrtille Camus at random. As he would choose another victim at random if he wasn't stopped. Myrtille Camus would still be alive if Captain Grima hadn't been blinded by his ridiculous hypothesis that Morgane's murder was an accident. An aberration committed by a respectable boy who had panicked and gripped the throat of his one-night stand a bit too hard; a respectable boy who would never again . . .

Commander Bastinet's response was to invite Carmen to meet with him. He assured her that every resource had been put at his disposal.

It was true.

Judge Lagarde and Commander Bastinet cast their gigantic net over Normandy, conducting door-to-door inquiries, house searches, collecting witness statements, cross-referencing cases stored on the database. Bastinet wasn't anticipating a speedy resolution. He thought it would be a lengthy investigation that would probe every minute detail in hope of finding some vital clue buried among the countless gigabytes of information . . . The same work that Captain

Grima had done in Fécamp, basically, but with many times the funding.

Ellen Nilsson, the criminal psychologist, was bored. Unlike Inspector Bastinet, she was staking everything on a single witness statement. Just one.

She seized upon the fundamental difference between the murder of Morgane Avril and that of Myrtille Camus.

Myrtille Camus had felt threatened during the days leading up to her murder.

And her family knew who she felt threatened by.

I looked up. I had almost finished reading, but the presence of a familiar silhouette on the beach, about a hundred metres away from me, made me lose my place.

Xanax!

He was still wearing his brown jacket like a second skin. He looked so weary and depressed, it was a wonder he hadn't thrown himself from the cliff. He was slowly walking towards the sea, almost as if he was waiting for the shoreline to dry behind the retreating waves.

Everyone was clearing out, even the sea.

That must have been part of his neurosis.

I hurriedly bundled the papers into the envelope and ran towards him.

As one of the three witnesses to Magali Verron's suicide, I wondered what he made of this unlikely sequence of coincidences. Whether he too believed that the red-scarf killer had struck again, ten years after claiming his first two victims.

14

Is he going to start again?

'Christian? Christian Le Medef?'

I walked as quickly as I could over the rocks exposed by the departing tide. A desert landscape after a miraculous rain shower. Thousands of miniature peaks, valleys and caves dug by the wind and the years. Sharp. Gleaming. My left foot caught on a ridge, slipped in a furrow. I cursed inwardly. If I wasn't capable of keeping my balance on a slippery shoreline with my wonky foot, it wasn't even worth me lining up with the others on the snowy slopes of Mont Blanc.

I called out again.

'Le Medef!'

Xanax turned around this time and stared at me with his weary eyes.

'Ah, It's you.'

Apparently he couldn't remember my name. I walked over to him and shook his hand.

'Jamal. Jamal Salaoui.'

He studied my WindWall. The one I had worn the previous day and all the other mornings.

'So you go running every day?'

'Yeah . . .'

I didn't want to go into detail about my training. I looked for some way of broaching the topic of Magali Verron's suicide.

'I'm due to see the police at Fécamp again this afternoon. I have a two o'clock meeting. And you?'

Le Medef looked surprised. 'I signed my statement yesterday. Captain Piroz said he would contact me again if necessary but he thought he had everything he needed for the time being . . . I'm not going to complain.'

He looked around him, and I wondered if he was pondering the daily training regime that had brought me along the cliff path. From the base of the cliff, the rocky shoreline seemed to stretch out endlessly. A vast wilderness populated only by the black, bent shadows of locals collecting shellfish. Several dozen of them, in scattered groups of two or three.

'It's forbidden,' Le Medef told me.

'What is?'

'Collecting shellfish. It's forbidden. There's a sign posted by the first aid post, and yet everyone does it. The cops don't say anything. It's beyond me . . .'

He raised his voice, perhaps in the hope of being heard by the foragers.

'Either it's dangerous and you impose the law, or it isn't and you let these good people pick their mussels. But forbidding something while tolerating it at the same time – there's nothing more hypocritical than that, is there?'

'I don't know. I've never collected shellfish.'

'You don't think the police are hypocritical?'

'Criminal, if you ask me!'

I pulled a face, communicating my disgust at the very idea of eating a sticky mollusc that's been pulled off a rock after sitting in the sun for hours. That cheered Le Medef up. I realised that I'd shifted to calling him Le Medef; the incongruity of this beaten-down individual sharing a name with the bosses' union tickled me.

'So that's how it is,' he said. 'Captain Piroz wants to see you again?'

'Yeah.'

'It's logical, I suppose . . . Me and Denise – not to mention good old Arnold – didn't really see anything. Just the girl crashing to the ground. Whereas you had a balcony seat.'

His eyes seemed drawn once again by the shell-pickers.

'Imagine if they were all poisoned, Jamal. If they all died. Or just one of them. An old one. Or a child. After eating a crab or a lobster crammed with bacteria. Given that we're here, between the oil refinery and the nuclear plant, the possibility isn't too far-fetched.'

Every now and again we heard shouts from the nearest group of shell-pickers, fifty metres away: a grandfather and his two grandchildren. Boots, yellow waxed jackets and a Hello Kitty pail.

No, I wasn't imagining it.

'Weird business, isn't it?' Le Medef resumed.

I worked out that he was talking about Magali Verron again.

'How do you mean?'

'Captain Piroz told you, I suppose. The cops don't think it was suicide. The kid was raped, then strangled. But your version is slightly different, isn't it?'

I had no time to reply, he'd already picked up the conversation again.

'I have to say, your version surprised me – the girl jumping off the cliff of her own accord. So I did some research into this Magali Verron.'

He leaned towards me and lowered his voice. He was standing in a hole filled with salt water in his unsuitable footwear, but he didn't seem to notice.

'I found some things. Some things that were hard to believe . . . I spent a while looking; I don't have much else to do with my time.'

'What do you mean?'

'I'm unemployed, divorced, I rarely see my children, now they're away at university . . .'

I'd been asking what he'd found out about Magali Verron, but now he was giving me his life story. I was wondering how to get him back on track without seeming rude when he brought his stubbly chin close to my shoulder.

'I was working at the nuclear plant in Paluel. High-ranking engineer! It's not easy, you know, particularly when you're a bit of an ecologist. Eight years ago, I gave it all up to invest in wind turbines. They were the future! My wife was OK with it – she's a bit green as well. Or rather, she was. So I set up my own company, even took on two technicians and a marketing person, we were going to go around all the farmers in the area to sell them wind . . . That stupid name of mine, Le Medef, had never been so appropriate.'

He let out a laugh. I didn't join in. His stale aftershave mingled with the sea spray. His voice assumed a melodramatic tone. A little too forced, but at the time I didn't give it much thought. It was only later, much later, that it came back to me.

'Next thing I know, all the big companies are getting in on the act,' Le Medef huffed. 'Nordex. Veolia. Suez. Then they introduce a new law banning the installation of wind turbines on land belonging to private individuals. Not a single pylon could be set up without a public utility investigation and a revision of the town planning scheme. I won't give you chapter and verse, but all the small companies melted away within six months, leaving the multinationals to carve up the cake. I had to declare myself bankrupt! My wife ran off with the guy who had taken my old job at the plant. I found myself up to my eyeballs in debt to pay for my kids' education. Every month I get bills for repayment of those loans, but all I get from my kids is a postcard once a year – if I'm lucky.'

Le Medef reminded me of the guys you find on sitting benches in the Cité des 4000. Sit down next to them and they'll give you their whole life story. As if just by telling it to you they can offload their misery.

'A year ago,' he went on, 'I became homeless. Luckily I met an old man who needed someone to do a bit of work on his house in Yport. He let me stay in his holiday home. He never goes there, but he doesn't want to sell it. I do some repairs, I mow the lawn, I maintain the place, and in return he lets me stay there for nothing. I'm waiting here until things pick up again. I can't complain – there are a lot worse places I could be.'

Like a swimmer running out of air, he paused to draw breath. I made a show of checking my watch. As I'd hoped, it didn't go unnoticed.

'Anyway, to get back to the subject of Magali Verron: did Piroz talk to you about her?'

'He told me she was a pharmaceutical sales rep, that she was

111

meeting with doctors in the area. That she had probably slept in Yport, but they don't know where . . .'

Le Medef turned towards the kids and their grandfather again. His face had taken on a concerned expression, as if they were in mortal danger.

'He told me much the same, but I did some digging. At the Paluel nuclear plant, I worked with the local hospitals, and the doctors too. Checking air quality, the distribution of dosimeters and iodine tablets, the whole thing. I called a few of my old contacts. They all knew the Verron girl. Quite a hottie, from the sound of it! She worked for Bayer France. They all described her as attractive, efficient, and flirtatious enough for them to order drugs from her. You saw her better than I did. A beautiful girl like that, if she'd recommended anti-radiation hallucinogenic mushrooms they'd have ordered them by the pallet. By all accounts, she was a perfectly ordinary girl . . . Apparently.'

Le Medef had the gift of drawing things out to keep his audience in suspense.

'Why "apparently"?'

He stepped towards the rocks. A dark line had appeared at the bottom of his shoes.

'My pumps are wet! I'm going back to the village. Will you come with me?'

I stayed right where I was. 'What have you found out about Magali Verron?' I demanded. 'That she *wasn't* a perfectly ordinary girl?'

'Follow me,' he insisted. 'You have to be in the village to understand . . .'

I had no choice. I caught up with him. As we walked towards the sea wall it occurred to me that Christian Le Medef had lived in the region for more than ten years. He must have made the connection between Magali Verron's suicide and the murders of Morgane Avril and Myrtille Camus. The red scarf . . . I thought about broaching that topic, but in the end I opted to walk with him in silence.

One revelation after another . . .

We passed the Sirène and Le Medef turned on to Rue Emmanuel-Foy, Yport's shopping street.

'You'll see,' he said. 'It's incredible!'

He came to a halt outside the newsagent.

'Look at the papers on the display stand,' he urged.

I studied the headlines of *Paris-Normandie*, *Le Havre Presse*, *Le Courrier Cauchois*. I didn't notice anything particular. I turned to Le Medef.

'I . . . I don't see anything.'

'Exactly. Don't you see? That's what's so odd. A girl jumps off the cliff, probably raped, strangled. And the next day there's no mention of it in the local dailies.'

I understood then what Le Medef was getting at, but nevertheless I put forward an argument:

'But it's a suicide. It doesn't warrant front-page headlines.'

I stood aside for a man who was leaving the shop with a copy of *L'Équipe* under his arm. The front page of *Le Courrier Cauchois* carried a story about the extension of the urban community of Fécamp, *Le Havre Presse* had a report on job losses in Port-Jérôme, *Paris-Normandie* was bemoaning the increase in house prices along the coast.

'Not on the front page?' Le Medef replied, raising his voice. 'Don't tell me you haven't made the connection. You've talked to people locally, haven't you? You know what's going on, for heaven's sake. That bloody serial killer is back! A rape, a girl strangled with a scarf that cost more than I get in benefits each month! Damn it, it was ten years ago and I remember it as if it was yesterday. The case made the front pages of all the papers for six months. And now? nothing! Nothing at all!'

'It's still quite recent,' I suggested. 'It only happened yesterday morning.'

'Exactly. Dear Christ! What a scoop! How could they miss it!'

I studied the front pages of the daily papers in the hope of finding at least a paragraph or two. Le Medef, sure of himself, let me get on with it. He must already have been through all the papers.

I tried to come up with another explanation.

'It's the police. They haven't let anything get out. They're waiting. A bit like when there's an accident at a nuclear plant – they don't say anything at first, they wait for the danger to pass before informing people.'

Le Medef didn't look convinced.

'And how would the cops have held on to the information? They've already got three witnesses. Since then I've talked to all my friends. You must have talked about it with people, right? Denise, too, she's the type. Not to mention all the people who saw the police on the beach yesterday, examining the body . . . And no one has said anything? In a village like Yport, where nothing ever happens and where the old people have nothing to do but spread gossip?'

Christian Le Medef was right. There was no way the newspapers wouldn't have received at least a few tip-offs. And local reporters would surely have spotted the parallels with the Avril–Camus investigation ten years earlier. That no one apart from us knew anything

. . .

And yet this seemed to be the case.

'So?' Le Medef pressed. 'Do you have an explanation?'

I shook my head.

'Neither do I. Believe me, young man, this whole business stinks.'

I realised that he had called me by the familiar *tu*, as if he was trying to establish a complicity between us in the middle of an inquiry that went beyond both of us. He looked away and pointed at a little fisherman's cottage. Blue shutters, red-brick walls decorated with flint, slate roof. As he'd said, it wasn't the worst emergency accommodation for a homeless man.

'This is my gaff! Would you like a coffee?'

Time was running out. I had less than three hours before my appointment with Piroz.

'No. I'm sorry. Do you happen to know where Denise lives?'

Christian Le Medef seemed disappointed.

'Probably with Arnold . . .' He smiled to himself. 'Apart from that, no idea. I haven't seen her since yesterday. I don't even know her surname, I'm afraid . . . And you're staying with André Jozwiak, at the Sirène?'

'Yes. For a week.'

'OK. If I find anything out, I'll let you know. I'm going to keep on digging, see what else I can find out about Magali Verron. Break the *omertà*, if you see what I mean. Last night I had Dr Charrier on the phone – he has a surgery in Doudeville, he's one of the doctors that Magali Verron visited before she went off the cliff. You see? Someone else who knows about this news story! Anyway, when it comes to women, Charrier isn't the kind to be easily impressed. You should see his secretaries – gorgeous, the pair of them. Well, he fell for little Magali. Tried to get off with her – chatted her up, asked her what she liked doing. She told him she was into dancing, so he invited her to a club, thinking he could show her some of his moves. Only it turned out the lovely Magali wasn't into disco, she did modern oriental dance – *raqs sharqi*, that kind of thing.

Raqs sharqi . . .

An electric shock exploded in my brain. The neurones tried in vain to reconnect.

Christian Le Medef went on talking, probably imagining Magali Verron in a spangled sari, his doctor friend drooling from the sidelines.

I wasn't listening to him any more.

I waved at him briefly.

'See you soon, Christian. Keep me up to date with your research.'

The Sirène was barely a hundred metres away. I tried not to run.

Raqs sharqi.

No sign of André at reception. I climbed the hotel steps, opened the window, then ran towards my laptop and turned it on, cursing its slowness in advance. The Windows wheel rotated more slowly than my thoughts.

Raqs sharqi

I had read that phrase for the first time the previous day in one of the brown envelopes.

In the biographical note on Morgane Avril!

While my computer whirred, I spread out all the pages about

Morgane Avril's life on the bed. Press articles, police notes, interviews . . .

At last, the arrow on my screen indicated that we were ready to go.

I feverishly typed in the name.

Magali Verron

A dozen results appeared.

Facebook. Copains d'avant. Twitter. LinkedIn. Dailymotion.

I picked up a piece of paper. With the first pen that came to hand I drew a line. One column for Magali, one for Morgane. I jotted down the information that I found, then arranged it in order of importance.

Date and place of birth, schools attended, musical tastes, leisure, countries visited . . .

Soon the list of words and names filled both sides of the page.

I searched again until there was no more information available.

The lines danced in front of my eyes. Surreal.

Was Fate mocking me?

15

A girl with no past?

'Mona? Where are you?'

'Jamal? You're awake! I'm on my way back from Grainval, just approaching Yport now.'

'OK, I'll join you there. I need to talk to you, the sooner the better. Something weird has come up.'

'Something to do with your serial killer?'

'More to do with his victims.'

When I reached the sea wall, a voice called to me.

'Jamal, I'm over here!'

Mona.

She was sitting on a swing in the children's playground overlooking the beach. A slide. A little climbing wall. A rope bridge. She was swaying gently, as if to dry the neoprene wetsuit that was open to her chest. By her feet she had put a rucksack containing a selection of pebbles that could revolutionise the computer industry.

As I approached, one detail threw me completely. Mona was wearing my sheriff's star pinned to her wetsuit. It confirmed my decision: she was the one person I could share my insane theory with.

I sat down facing her, on the edge of a miniature paddling pool that was only in use when the weather was fine, assuming it ever was around here. A copper fish, which was supposed to spit water into the basin, stared at us with its mouth open and empty.

'Well?' Mona asked me. 'What did you want to show me?'

I passed her the page, covered on both sides with my handwriting.

'Look, Mona! Two columns. One for Magali Verron, who died yesterday. One for Morgane Avril, murdered ten years ago. I made a note of everything I could find about them. Listen to this . . . Morgane Avril was a fan of seventies progressive rock bands like Pink Floyd, Yes, Genesis – it was in the police report. That was why she'd been so keen to go to the Riff on the Cliff festival. According to her Facebook page, Magali Verron belonged to some music fan clubs. Three, to be precise: Pink Floyd, Yes and Genesis.

'Along with a few thousand other fans, right?'

Mona's swing squeaked like a plaintive bird. I lowered my eyes towards my page.

'OK, I'll go on. Morgane was into *raqs sharqi*—'

'Oh, that's all the rage. It's like the Bollywood version of ballroom—'

'Magali was into *raqs sharqi* as well.'

'Like I was saying, it's all—'

'A coincidence? Wait for it, Mona; this is just the beginning. Morgane Avril attended the local public schools in Neufchâtel-en-Bray, between 1986 and 2003. I wrote down all the names: Charles Perrault nursery school, Claude Monet primary school, Albert Schweitzer middle school, Georges Brassens high school. Nothing out of the ordinary, and nothing to do with Magali Verron, who grew up in Val-de-Marne, south of Paris. After primary school, in September 2004, she attended middle school in Créteil . . . Guess the name of the school?'

By way of answer, the swing let out three more cries.

'Albert Schweitzer!'

Mona's swing deviated from its steady rhythm. Ignoring her startled expression, I went on:

'And here's another coincidence: Magali attended a high school twenty kilometres from Créteil, at Courcouronnes. And the name of that school was—'

'Georges Brassens?' Mona guessed.

'Precisely! I've checked, there are fewer than ten Lycées Georges

Brassens in France . . . Including one in Neufchâtel-en-Bray and one in Courcouronnes.'

'That's weird, granted, but—'

I ploughed on before she could finish:

'Then Morgane and Magali both studied medicine, Morgane in Rouen and Magali at Évry-Val-d'Essonne university.'

Morgane halted the swing with her foot.

'Were they related by any chance? Or friends?'

'No. I found no trace of Magali Verron in any of the articles and files on the Avril case. Besides, Magali was only ten when Morgane was murdered. And she didn't live in Normandy.'

The sea wind continued to move the swing which Mona had just got off. A cold wind. She pulled the zip of her wetsuit up to her neck. The star gleamed over her heart. 'OK,' she said. 'You're right on one point: this can't all be coincidence. So there has to be some kind of connection between the two girls . . . As far as we can tell, Morgane didn't know Magali Verron. Magali was ten years younger. She lived in Île de France.'

She frowned, wrinkling her little nose. Suddenly her eyes flashed with inspiration.

'On the other hand, even though she was only ten at the time, Magali must have heard of the Avril case and the red-scarf killer. The story might have triggered some form of trauma that made her identify with Morgane, copy her tastes, her hobbies, even down to her choice of middle school, then a high school with the same name as the one attended by Morgane Avril . . .'

I pulled a sceptical face.

'And then, ten years later, she gets herself raped, same as Morgane? Simulates strangulation with a Burberry scarf? Throws herself off a cliff?'

Mona took a deep breath. 'Hard to believe, I grant you.'

I drew closer to Mona. For a moment all I could think of was huddling against her wetsuit and opening the zip, but instead I went on:

'That's not all, Mona. It wasn't only Morgane Avril's death that Magali Verron copied.' I lowered my voice: 'She was born on 10

May 1993 – ten years to the day after Morgane Avril.'

'Morgane was born on 10 May 1983?'

'Yes, at the Fernand-Langlois hospital in Neufchâtel-en-Bray.'

Mona hiccupped.

'And where . . . where was Magali Verron born?'

'Nearly six thousand kilometres away, in the northern suburbs of Quebec . . .'

I gave Mona time to breathe, a long exhalation of relief, before dropping my next bombshell:

'I'll let you guess the name of the suburb . . .'

Her answer came slowly, as if stuck in her throat.

'Neufchâtel?'

'Yes! As incredible as it might seem, she was born in Neufchâtel, a village between Charlesbourg and Loretteville.'

Every muscle in Mona's face went slack, as if she had given up trying to make sense of it all. She took a step towards me and pressed her neoprene against my WindWall. The contact felt strange, as if we were two cosmonauts on Mars.

'Magali Verron didn't just copy Morgane Avril's death,' I repeated. 'She copied her birth. I've checked: in the entire world there are only five villages called Neufchâtel – four in France and one in Canada. Magali Verron arrived in France at the age of seven.'

'Damn it, Jamal, what the hell's going on?'

'I don't know, Mona. I have no idea. We're missing something. There must be a rational explanation.'

Still holding her close, I murmured in her ear: 'Copying someone else's life. Every stage, from start to finish. Their taste in music, dance, the places they went to – like a mirror, but from a distance. A kind of hologram. Hell, it's impossible!'

'A serial killer looks for victims who resemble one another, right?' said Mona, trying to apply logic, but without any real conviction. 'Maybe the two girls reminded him of his mother, his ex, or some—'

'But the killer didn't have to go looking for her, Mona! It's as if Magali Verron tried to turn herself into his prey, trying to lure the predator – until he found her . . .'

'Until she finished the job herself,' Mona added. 'Until she wrapped the murder weapon around her own neck. The last act of her life.'

I didn't reply. For a few seconds I listened to the waves washing over the pebbles, then I gently placed a kiss on her lips and ran my hand over her curves. As my hand went down to her hips, Mona's breathing quickened. I felt a swelling in the thin pocket of her wetsuit. My fingers explored it until I removed a yellow silk scarf.

'For my hair,' Mona murmured. 'A precaution against the Normandy weather.'

The scarf slipped through my fingers. Without even thinking about it, I raised my hands and held the scrap of fabric under her chin.

Slowly.

'How long would it take you to tie this thing?'

I brought the silk square to her neck again. A moment later, Mona's eyes blurred.

I read the fear in them. A sudden and intense terror, on the brink of the void.

Idiot!

I immediately lowered my arms, but the damage was done.

Her voice was thick with tears.

'Please, Jamal, don't play that game—'

'I'm sorry,' I sputtered. I didn't mean—'

She pulled the yellow scarf from my hand.

'Forget it. I'm the one who should be apologising, it was stupid of me to react that way.'

She took a moment to look at the fabric in the hollow of her palm.

'You know what I think, Jamal?'

'What's that?'

'It isn't possible.'

She stared at the cliff in front of us, the blockhouse, the sheep, the exact spot where Magali had fallen the previous day, and said it again.

'It's impossible for a girl falling from up there to be able to do that. To tie a scarf around her neck.'

She briskly brought both hands together, then ran them behind her head and rolled the yellow fabric around the back of her neck.

How long had it taken? Less than a second?

'It's not a matter of time, Jamal!' Mona said. 'It may be possible – technically. But can you imagine? Doing that while dropping like a stone from the top of a cliff. To focus on tying a scarf while ignoring everything else – it's impossible, Jamal. And yet I believe you: Magali didn't have that scarf around her neck at the top of the cliff, but she had it on when she landed at the bottom.'

'There . . . there must be a rational explanation.'

'Jamal, you've already said that.'

I fell silent. She was right. None of this made sense.

And yet . . .

Mona put the scarf back in her pocket. She sat down on the miniature rocking motorbike on springs and looked at me like a nurse reasoning with an uncooperative patient.

'To sum up what we know so far, Jamal: in 2004, a serial killer rapes and kills two women, Morgane Avril and Myrtille Camus. Ten years later, a girl dies in identical circumstances. Two hypotheses. First the twisted hypothesis: the girl was recreating every aspect of Morgane Avril's life, her musical tastes, her schools, her hobbies . . . Even taking her own life in a way that mimicked her death.'

'And choosing the same date and place of birth as Morgane,' I added. 'No way!'

'No way – we agree. So let's move on to the second, more logical hypothesis. The killer strikes again, but at random this time – given all that we know about Magali Verron. He chooses his victim, he rapes and strangles her. That's more or less the police theory, isn't it?'

'But that doesn't fit either! Magali wasn't strangled, she committed suicide.'

Mona nodded gently and remained thoughtful for a few moments.

'Except,' I went on, 'I've got a meeting with Captain Piroz in less than two hours and, to tell you the truth, Mona, I'm scared shitless. I . . . I look a bit too much like the perfect suspect . . .'

'They can't frame you – it's not your sperm, Jamal! Do you have a record?'

'No!'

'You've never killed anybody? You've never stolen?'

She rocked gently on the motorbike. In her latex wetsuit, with her hair down over her shoulders, she looked like a Hell's Angel on a toy Harley.

'Yes, I stole – to pay for my studies. But I never got caught, I had an infallible method.'

Her eyes gleamed. She was clearly happy to change the subject.

'Another one?'

'I only stole in the summer, by the rivers, in the gorges of the Tarn or the Ardèche. You know, those canoe and kayak highways. I helped myself directly from the tubs where tourists left their papers, watches and mobile phones, particularly in the sites where they left their boats on the shore to jump from the rocks. At the campsite or on the beach, it was impossible to go through people's bags because everyone keeps an eye on everyone else. But put on a yellow life jacket and wander among thirty identical canoes – no one pays you any attention.'

Mona nearly fell off her motorbike.

'Christ! That's a brilliant scam! You really did that?'

She studied every inch of my face.

'Perhaps . . . I love making up stories.'

'And the red scarf, did you make that up too?'

That had slipped out. She had added it automatically. At least, that was what I thought at that moment, that it hadn't been premeditated.

My face closed.

'Damn it, not you too, Mona!'

'What do you mean, "not you too"?'

'Mona, listen to me, I'm would never joke about stuff like that. That girl was murdered. Raped. I thought you knew me better than that, Mona. If I can't trust you, who can I trust?'

I looked her straight in the eyes before continuing:

'If I can't trust you, who can I trust?'

She seemed hurt. She got to her feet and tried not to raise her voice as I had done.

'It's fine, Jamal. Calm down. I believe you.'

My heart was pounding. I hadn't been bluffing. There was no one else I could turn to. It was impossible to face this madness all on my own.

If Mona left me . . .

If Mona left me, who would believe me?

The police?

André? Christian Le Medef? Denise and Arnold?

You?

16

One more coincidence?

The silence between Mona and me could have lasted an eternity. The riff from 'La Grange' by ZZ Top exploded before she could disappear.

The alert on my phone! I'd received a message. Irritably, I took the phone from the depths of my pocket.

'An admirer?' Mona asked curiously.

She seemed delighted that something had intervened to break the spider's web in which we had become entangled. I read the message and opted for appeasement.

'You don't know how right you are . . .'

'Young and pretty?'

'Pretty, yes. But very young.'

'How old?'

'Fifteen.'

Mona stood on tiptoes and looked at me with astonishment.

'Her first name is Ophélie. She's a pupil at the Saint Antoine Institute. She was raped by her father. A present for her eighth birthday. It had certain consequences. Violence. Behavioural difficulties. Sexual problems . . . No adult, social worker, shrink or teacher could get to the root of it. But the two of us get on.'

'She calls you on holiday?'

'Yes. The Institute have given me a hard time, they say I'm too close to her, that I'm disrupting her therapy—'

'They're right,' Mona said 'Everybody has his job to do, right? What does the girl want?'

I held out the phone to Mona to show her the photograph that Ophélie had sent. She was posing pressed up against a tall black guy with a piercing that covered half of one nostril. There was a short message under the photograph. Two words.

What mark??

'What does she mean, "What mark"?'

I took back the telephone.

'It's a game we play. At the weekend or on holiday, when Ophélie picks up a guy, she sends me a picture of him and I appraise him . . . I grade him, if you like. Along the lines of: "Could do better", "Making progress", "Out of the question". In return, I sometimes send her photographs of my girlfriends . . .'

Mona, reassured, burst out laughing.

'And you're surprised that the social workers at the Institute come down on you like a ton of bricks?'

I quickly typed in my reply.

5 out of 20. Lack of imagination. Avoid copying and pasting.

While I was clicking to send the message, Mona suddenly opened her wetsuit, defying the wind that swept between the sea wall and the beach huts. Her breasts came delicately away from the neoprene.

'And what mark do I get?'

This girl was crazy!

'You want my friend's opinion, is that it?'

I zoomed my iPhone in on Mona's face.

'It's gone. Brace yourself. Ophélie is a tough cookie. So far she's given no more than an average mark to any of my girlfriends.'

I took a step towards Mona.

'Get dressed before you catch your death. I'm off, I have to go back to the cops.'

I pulled the zip so that Mona's plunging neckline turned into a respectable polo neck.

I had time to drop by at the hotel to change, and then grab a sandwich before taking the bus to Fécamp for my appointment at the police station.

As I entered the lobby of the Sirène, André was rearranging the display of leaflets advertising local attractions. He was forever appearing and disappearing from behind his counter, as if he had a trapdoor under the bar.

It didn't look as though he had any new mail for me . . . I went and stood in front of him.

'André, can you recall having a guest by the name of Magali Verron? She was a pharmaceutical sales rep who dealt with a lot of the local surgeries. She must have checked into hotels when she was in the area. The day before yesterday, for example.'

'Is that the girl who committed suicide?'

He went on indifferently arranging the brochures: Étretat Vélo-Rail, Musée des Terre-Neuvas. I fought the urge to ask how he had made the connection so quickly.

'Yes.'

'Doesn't ring a bell. You know, there are a dozen hotels in the area, not counting the ones around Étretat, and then there's all the farmhouse bed and breakfasts. Have you got a photograph?'

'No.'

I tried to describe Magali Verron as best I could: her beauty, the seductive power of her desperate eyes.

'I'd have noticed a girl as pretty as that,' said André.

Indeed.

As I climbed the wooden stairs, my phone vibrated.

A new message.

Ophélie's response to Mona's photograph . . .

I read the text, convinced that my little protégée would deliver a jealous and scathing critique. Her message left me speechless:

127

When I opened the door to my room, I was caught off guard by the icy draught. The window had been left open.

The housekeeper. To air the room.

The bed had been made. New towels laid out. I thought for a moment of the chaos of the room after the night I had spent with Mona.

Then I froze.

There was a brown envelope on my desk, just beside my laptop. A new, unopened envelope. No stamp this time. No address. Just my name.

Jamal Salaoui.

The same female handwriting as on the previous packages.

Before picking up the envelope, I leaned out the window. The gust of wind froze my overheated body. It wasn't very hard to get to my room from outside; the flat roofs of the restaurant of the Sirène and its outbuildings formed a kind of staircase for a giant. But who would have risked such a climb? Right on the seafront, in full view of everybody? To put an envelope on my desk.

For a moment I thought of going back downstairs and asking André whether, apart from the housekeeper, anybody had visited my room. I thought better of it.

Later, perhaps . . .

I closed the window. I had to calm down. My WindWall was supposed to absorb perspiration, but rivulets of sweat were running down my body. I got undressed on the bed and unscrewed my carbon prosthesis. My hands were damp. They left brown traces on the envelope as I tore it open. It was thinner than the others. Just three stapled sheets of paper.

I immediately recognised the tricolour letterhead of the police:

Caen Police Department: Myrtille Camus case
Statement, 28 August 2004
Item no. 027: Witness statement by Alina Masson

Naked on the bed but for my boxer shorts, I let my one leg dangle to the floor as I tried to control the nervous tremors running through it.

Myrtille Camus case – Saturday, 28 August 2004

'I was Myrtille's best friend.'

'We know,' Bastinet replied.

The commander of Caen police and the criminal psychologist Ellen Nilsson sat facing the four witnesses. Louise and Charles, the parents of Myrtille Camus. Frédéric Saint-Michel, her fiancé. Alina Masson, her best friend, who had just spoken.

Whose statement would prove to be crucial . . .

Commander Bastinet didn't need to consult his notes, he knew the file by heart. Since the girl's body had been discovered, he'd had less than five hours' sleep, snatched in half-hour blocks, as if he were a navigator taking part in a rally. That was what it felt like.

A race.

Against the clock.

To catch the bastard who had already struck twice in three months. Morgane Avril in Yport, in June, and now Myrtille Camus.

To tell the truth, he didn't attach much value to the contribution of Ellen Nilsson, the girl the ministry had lumbered him with. Not that he had anything against criminal psychologists; in the past he had often sought their advice in the hope of gaining a better understanding of the lunatics he had to deal with. But he wondered how this blonde – who had turned up with her Dupont pen case as her only weapon, her Mont Blanc notepad as her only armour and her Activia yoghurt as her only source of nourishment – could be of any use to him.

'Mademoiselle Masson, you ran the camp for teenagers where Myrtille Camus was killed?'

Aline nodded.

Practically a child herself! Bastinet thought.

Alina Masson was twenty-one, a few months older than Myrtille Camus. In the Cloth of Gold camp at Isigny-sur-Mer, there was no hierarchy between the two girls. Just an enduring friendship.

Bastinet decided to get straight to the point.

'Did Myrtille feel threatened? Threatened by a man, on several occasions? Is that so, Mademoiselle Masson?'

'Not exactly, Commander.'

Bastinet raised an eyebrow.

Ellen Nilsson, studying her emerald-green fingernails, tried a different approach. 'Take your time, Mademoiselle Masson. Tell us the facts. Just the facts. Who was this man?'

'The first time I saw him,' Alina explained, 'was by the pond at Isigny leisure centre. He was standing about a hundred metres away from us. He . . . he was staring at Myrtille.'

'What was your reaction?' Bastinet asked.

'None. At that point I wasn't really paying attention. It happened, how can I put it, frequently.'

'Frequently?' Bastinet repeated.

Alina glanced awkwardly at Frédéric Saint-Michel. Myrtille's fiancé gestured to her to continue. Ellen scribbled some notes on her Mont Blanc pad while Commander Bastinet urged the witness to continue.

'Every morning Myrtille led a half-hour aqua aerobics session at the pool. We put on some loud music, Myrtille danced and all the kids would join in. Within a few days, the whole campsite was joining in. Families, tourists, teenagers . . .'

'All eyes were on her,' Ellen suggested.

'Right.' Alina hesitated, glanced quizzically at Louise Camus, then went on, with a nervous tremor in her voice. 'Myrtille was a very pretty girl. She danced with such grace and energy that everyone loved to watch.'

Tears welled up in the corners of Louise's eyes. The former dance teacher gripped her husband's wrinkled hand.

'Can you give us a description of this man who was staring at Myrtille?' Bastinet cut in. 'This man who was staring at her more than the rest.'

'I only saw him in the distance, Commander. Average height. Quite young. Our age, I would say. He was wearing a cap, white and blue, with the three Adidas stripes. Sunglasses too. He seemed quite tanned.'

Bastinet cursed. The description could easily have matched the stranger with the red scarf spotted by three witnesses in Yport, the number one suspect in the murder of Morgane Avril, the one that Captain Grima had looked for in vain. But it could also have matched thousands of other men.

'When did you see this man again?'

'He hung around at the campsite, or at least I recognised his cap a few times. I assumed he must be local. Either that or a camp leader for one of the other groups at the base. There were at least ten camps in Isigny at that time . . .'

'Seven,' Bastinet corrected her. 'One hundred and thirteen teenagers and twenty-eight adults in charge of them.'

Ellen Nilsson raised her eyes to the sky, as if wearied by Bastinet's manner.

'To be precise,' Alina continued, 'the second time I noticed him was off Saint-Marcouf.'

Bastinet consulted his notes. The Îles Saint-Marcouf, seven kilometres off the Normandy coast, were two little rocks set in the sea, on which Napoleon had built a fort against the British. They were state property, overnight stays were forbidden, but mooring was permitted. They were a favourite destination of the local sailing clubs. The Cloth of Gold group had booked a boat trip to the islands, five days before Myrtille's murder.

'Myrtille and the five teenagers in her care spent the day on the archipelago,' Alina went on. 'I came and joined them with another group at about midday. I . . . I spotted the guy: same cap, same sunglasses. He was on a Zodiac, a small model, it looked like a rental boat. And he was sailing around the islands.

'How long had he been doing that?' Ellen asked.

'I don't know . . . He was already there when we arrived at Saint-Marcouf. He sailed around the island a few more times. It was obvious he was staring at Myrtille. Then he opened the throttle and roared off. It couldn't have gone on more than five minutes in all, but—'

'But this time,' Bastinet cut in, 'it worried you.'

Ellen sighed heavily.

'Not exactly, Commander,' Alina explained. 'I thought something along the lines of: he's starting to get on my nerves, hanging around us like that.'

'I get it. As a vigilant team leader, you were naturally concerned. When did you last run into this man?'

'Two days later. Myrtille had the day off and was going to walk to the beach at Grandcamp-Maisy. We'd agreed that I would pick her up when I went shopping in the minibus. I arrived at the time we'd arranged and looked for her on the beach. She was asleep, in her swimming costume, lying on her back, with a scarf over her eyes. I woke her up. It was only then that I noticed he was there, on a towel, about thirty metres away. On the way back, Myrtille admitted she'd slept like a log for over two hours . . .' Her trembling fingers rummaged in her pocket for a handkerchief. She didn't find one, gave up and went on. 'So the guy could have been watching her all that time, imagining what he wanted to do, he could have . . .'

Alina fell suddenly silent and burst into tears. Frédéric Saint-Michel, hands clenched on the arms of her chair, didn't move to comfort her. It was as if it was all he could do to contain his hatred of his fiancée's killer, listening to this account of the moment when the voyeur's obsession might have turned into a murderous impulse.

While Ellen held out a tissue to Alina, Bastinet pressed on.

'Can you describe him to us?'

Alina sniffed, coughed to clear her throat, and shook her head. 'Not really. He was lying on his belly. Still with his cap on his head and his sunglasses. He was quite slender, quite muscular, with long muscles, like an athlete's. But I wouldn't be able to recognise him.'

The police then showed her the photofit picture of the Yport stranger, but with the red scarf photoshopped out and replaced by an Adidas cap, and with the addition of sunglasses.

It might have been him.

Or not.

Commander Bastinet smiled understandingly.

'OK, Mademoiselle Masson. There's one last thing I'd like to ask, which isn't meant for you alone. Do any of you happen to know if Myrtille kept a diary?'

'Not exactly, Commander. Not a diary as such.'

Parents, fiancé and friend took turns to describe the sky-blue Moleskine notebook that Myrtille had written in since her teenage years, and which she always kept on her person or in her handbag.

Both had disappeared, presumably into the hands of her rapist.

Myrtille entrusted her most secret thoughts to that notebook. A few lines a day, sometimes funny, sometimes melancholy. Myrtille loved to write.

Bastinet was about to thank the four witness when Ellen raised her hand. The criminal psychologist had been hesitant about asking her last question in front of Myrtille Camus's fiancé. Perhaps it was the age gap between Frédéric Saint-Michel and his future wife that troubled her, though at the age of thirty-seven he still possessed a charismatic charm, combining the gentle expression of a Buddhist monk with the build of a black belt in judo.

Ellen adopted the calmest voice she could muster, and then spoke directly to Alina.

'Mademoiselle Masson, in your view, on the day of the murder, why was Myrtille Camus dressed so elegantly?'

Aline froze, surprised. 'What do you mean?'

Ellen held up an emerald finger (ring and fingernail coordinated) to warn Bastinet not to intervene, and went on:

'Myrtille was an activity leader at a camp for teenagers. Under your direction. I assume she wore practical clothes for work – shorts, a T-shirt, trainers . . . Not mauve underwear and such a short dress.'

'It was . . . it was her day off,' Alina stammered, surprised that the criminal psychologist had forgotten.

Commander Bastinet glared at his colleague. Frédéric Saint-Michel clenched his hands on his chair to contain his rage. Louise and Charles calmly rose to their feet like silent ghosts.

The commander studied Frédéric Saint-Michel as he left the

room. Tall. Straight-backed. Still proud. His long hair tied in a ponytail. The months of mourning ahead would rob him of his youthful looks, thought Bastinet. Whether or not the murderer of his future wife was found, it wouldn't change a thing, Saint-Michel's long hair would turn white and he would shrivel with age.

Love stories have a tendency to end badly, Bastinet thought stupidly.

In the days that followed, Ellen Nilsson's question wormed its way into Alina Masson's mind. She couldn't stop thinking about that short dress, that mauve underwear.

Alina thought about returning to talk to Ellen Nilsson about it. Several times she picked up the phone, but she couldn't bring herself to dial the number on the card the criminal psychologist had given her. She didn't completely trust the smooth-faced shrink.

Even if she had gone straight to the heart of the matter.

She alone.

So Alina remained silent. She regretted it more with each passing day, but to express her doubts would be to betray Myrtille's secret. Her best, her only friend.

Charles and Louise Camus, meanwhile, drew closer to Carmen Avril.

Even though they were different in every respect, they combined their forces.

Charles and Louise wanted peace, Carmen wanted war.

Charles and Louise were inspired by a sense of justice, Carmen by a feeling of hatred.

But basically their goal was the same.

To know the truth.

To discover the identity of the murderer of Morgane Avril and Myrtille Camus

Commander Bastinet ordered his men to focus on the search for their number one suspect.

The man in the Adidas cap.

In response to the photofits distributed and posted in the area, a number of witnesses came forward to confirm what Alina Masson had told the police. The young man in the cap had been seen about the campsite in Isigny-sur-Mer, on the beach at Grandcamp-Maisy, around the sailing club . . .

Though they'd seen him . . . no one could identify him. He didn't work locally; the police checked with all employers in the area and none had hired anyone matching the description.

A solitary predator, blending in with the crowd of summer visitors?

The very fact that he didn't voluntarily turn up at a police station to give a statement further reinforced Commander Bastinet's conviction that this was the rapist-murderer. The same man who had worn that red scarf in Yport.

The more days that passed, the more Bastinet despaired of tracing the man. He had slipped through the net. They might never find out who he was, barring some huge stroke of luck. And Bastinet, from experience, didn't believe in luck.

He was wrong.

Fortune tipped in favour of the investigators two months later, on 3 November 2004, to be precise. The day when the police discovered the identity of the boy with the Adidas cap.

By then it was too late.

The Camus–Avril case had been overshadowed by two more deaths.

17

Fate tips the scales?

I almost missed the bus for Fécamp. I caught up with it at the intersection of Sente Colin and Rue Cramoisan. The driver had no hesitation in breaking the rules to let me on while the vehicle was still in motion – that was the advantage of running after a bus on one leg.

I spent the half-hour journey trying to sort things out in my head. Almost in spite of myself, I was obsessed by the incredible similarities between the suicide of Magali Verron and the murder of Morgane Avril ten years previously. That succession of coincidences that no police officer could swallow. But I was sure that I would also have to find out more about the murder of Myrtille Camus, the serial killer's second victim. If the stranger was sending me details of that investigation, it had to be for a reason. I would need to commit every clue to memory. It was all part of the same jigsaw puzzle, and if I was to find the solution I would have to slot every piece carefully in its place.

The bus dropped me in Fécamp, on Quai de la Vicomté, at 1.45 p.m. Just time to pick up a ham salad sandwich at the bakery opposite and eat it in the harbour, facing the sea wall. When I arrived at the police station I concealed my nerves by exchanging pleasantries with the receptionist who looked like an air hostess.

'I've been called in to see Piroz,' I said, like a schoolboy who's been summoned to see the headmaster.

The girl cop played the part of the sympathetic supervisor who's all too familiar with her boss's ill humour. She even managed a 'good luck' before I stepped into the corridor.

At two o'clock on the dot I was standing outside Captain Piroz's office.

The door was open. I paused for barely a second.

'Come in, Monsieur Salaoui.'

Piroz gestured for me to close the door behind me. His grey hair, combed back, fell on his shoulders like the branches of a weeping willow with a coating of frost.

'Sit down.'

He didn't look like a headmaster who was about to read the riot act to a hopeless boy, more like a consultant who has no good news to pass on to his patient. The stack of files behind the model of the *Étoile-de-Noël* was growing.

'I've got your results, Monsieur Salaoui.'

Not just any old specialist. An oncologist.

'It doesn't look good, Monsieur Salaoui.'

'Meaning?'

'The fingerprints . . .' Piroz combed his greasy hair with his fingers. 'They're yours.'

Even though I'd been prepared for it, this was a hard blow to take.

'On the Burberry scarf?'

Piroz nodded.

'Let me explain, Captain.'

Piroz didn't interrupt me once while I told him my version of events, my discovery of the scarf caught on the barbed wire near the blockhouse, my idiotic reflex in throwing it to Magali Verron. Her leap into the void, the scarf floating from her hand. I had rehearsed what I would say on the bus, but I still stammered when I told him what had happened next.

The beach.

The scarf wrapped around the neck of the suicide.

I suggested the version put forward by Mona, that the girl hadn't seen her rapist's face, she'd confused me with him, she'd panicked,

137

she'd jumped to get away from me, to accuse me. I didn't believe it myself, but I did my best to sound sincere. I sensed that Piroz would take some convincing.

I was wide of the mark.

'Your version is interesting, Monsieur Salaoui. But you interrupted me a moment ago. The fingerprints are yours, on the red cashmere scarf, quite definitely . . .'

He opened the green file in front of him. From experience, I knew it wasn't a good sign.

'But you'll have to explain to me, Monsieur Salaoui, why we also found your fingerprints on Magali Verron's neck, on her legs and on her chest . . .'

I froze.

Paralysed.

My whole body was now as stiff as my left leg. I struggled to breathe.

'It's . . . it's impossible, Captain. I never touched the girl.'

Piroz looked up from his file and leaned his head back, as if the weight of his hair was pulling it down.

'You didn't touch her before she jumped, that's what you told me. But on the beach, when she was already dead?'

'I didn't touch her, Captain! Not before her death, and not afterwards either. Christian Le Medef and that old lady, Denise, must have told you that . . .'

'I'm just trying to help you, Monsieur Salaoui.'

Like hell he was.

I replayed the scene in my head, trying to remember every detail. There was no doubt in my mind. I had never been in direct contact with Magali Verron.

What was this new insanity?

'I don't believe in your nonsense for a second, Captain,' I sneered. 'What next? Are you going to tell me my sperm was in Magali Verron's vagina?'

Piroz calmly smoothed a grey curl between his thumb and his index finger.

'That would make a lot of sense, Monsieur Salaoui. The man

who strangled Magali Verron is probably the one who raped her.'

I exploded. The *Étoile-de-Noël* pitched and tossed in front of my eyes.

'Christ alive! I tried to save that girl! I tried to prevent her falling, and you're accusing me of . . .'

I didn't have the strength to finish. Piroz's smile chilled my blood. An even more intense fear pierced my heart.

He hadn't told me everything.

I spat out another question.

'Do you have the results of the DNA test? Is that it?'

'No . . . Not yet, perhaps this evening . . . But I've had the preliminary findings. They're not good. Not good for you!'

Christ almighty!

I was sitting in an electric chair that had just passed two thousand volts through my body. My sperm in Magali Verron's vagina . . . That was what that bastard was implying.

The policeman's calm contrasted with the storm that was blowing through my head.

'I think you already know what the outcome will be, Monsieur Salaoui. The examining magistrate signed your indictment this morning. There are still some formalities to sort out. You'll need to find yourself a lawyer, for example. But in the meantime, there are some things I would like to discuss with you.'

For the first time, there was a slight hesitation in his voice as he continued:

'I'd like to talk about the two murders that took place ten years ago: Morgane Avril and Myrtille Camus. Ten years ago. You remember, Monsieur Salaoui?'

Do I remember?

Suddenly I had the impression Piroz was on precarious ground, at the limit of what an examining magistrate would permit. I straightened up in my chair.

'Is that it, Captain? Three dead girls. You start by accusing me of killing the first one and then, while you're about it, you try to pin two more on me – crimes the police have been unable to solve for ten years.'

Piroz seemed unimpressed by my outburst.

'You must have carried out your own little investigation, Monsieur Salaoui. You must have noticed some striking similarities between the fate of Morgane Avril and that of Magali Verron. You're right, we're stuck . . . But there's at least one thing we're sure of: the three crimes are connected.'

I didn't trust myself to speak. I felt like a dog being restrained by the collar, ready to bite anyone who came within range.

'Explaining coincidences is your job, not mine.'

'True.' Piroz began delving through one of his files, a beige one, this time. 'I'm going to ask you an important question, Monsieur Salaoui. It's a simple enough question, and I'd like you to give me a straightforward answer. Did you still have the use of both legs ten years ago? Your file is a bit, shall we say, vague on this point.'

I had understood the implications without Piroz having to explain. The number one suspect in the Avril–Camus case, the stranger wearing a Burberry scarf, and perhaps three months later an Adidas cap, might vaguely match my description.

Dark-haired, average height, athletic, tanned.

Except he didn't have a limp . . .

Except nothing would induce me to tell Piroz the truth.

On this point at least.

'No, Captain. I was born like this . . . Well, almost. I was unlucky, the fairy who bent over my cradle had some sort of speech impediment.'

Piroz eyed me with suspicion. He'd scared me shitless with his accusations, but now it was time for me to have my revenge.

'That damned fairy waved her magic wand over my forehead, she said her magic word, abracadabra, or whatever, then she said, as true as I'm sitting here, Captain: "May this little boy be so blessed with gifts that when it comes to choosing one he's totally stumped."'

Piroz's expression was a picture.

'Just a slip of the tongue, Captain. Stupid, isn't it?'

The bubbles in my brain exploded like a firework display. I felt as if I was charging, sabre raised, at a tank.

Piroz turned brick red.

'This isn't a game, Salaoui. Damn it, I'm trying to help you.'

'Set me up, more like! A cripple. An Arab. Alone in the world. Working with loonies. The ideal scapegoat, don't you think? The police have been looking for one for ten years . . .'

Piroz placed both elbows on the desk.

I carried on: 'I didn't touch that girl, Captain. Those aren't my prints on her neck. It isn't my sperm. Find another fall guy!'

The policeman stared beyond the mizzen mast of the *Étoile-de-Noël* for a moment, then continued as calmly as possible:

'This isn't the right strategy, Salaoui. Your disability won't save you when you're up before a jury.'

Arsehole! So what is the right strategy?

When I'd reviewed it all in my mind earlier, I could come up with only one possible explanation.

A police conspiracy.

They needed someone to pin it on. Who better than the poor guy who happened to be on the cliff at the wrong time one morning?

Me.

A moment later, the other hemisphere of my brain whispered to me that I was at the police station in Fécamp, not in North Korea or South Africa . . . You didn't manufacture false evidence to trap an innocent party. Not here. Not in France . . .

'I have the right to see a lawyer.'

'Of course, Salaoui. It's impossible to put a citizen under examination before he has heard the accusations accompanied by a lawyer.'

Vague memories came back to me, of television series glimpsed from the battered sofa in our flat in La Courneuve. The kind of soporific crime shows my mother used to watch, and which I used to hang around in front of so as not to be sent to revise in my room.

The Avril–Camus case was almost ten years ago. Ten years, that must be the statute of limitation for murder cases.

What if I was their last throw of the dice?

The Avril–Camus case would be closed within a few months.

What if, before the final curtain came down, the police had decided to pin it on the first guy who came along?'

'Do you have a lawyer, Salaoui?'

I didn't answer. Something else had come to mind from one of my mother's favourite television series.

'Don't you need two police officers to interrogate somebody?'

'No, Monsieur Salaoui . . . Not for routine questioning.' Piroz got to his feet, clearly annoyed now. 'I have three detectives working the Magali Verron case, following up every lead, looking for all the guys she came across during her final days. They are also collating all the similarities and coincidences that link Magali Verron and Morgane Avril. You may not realise it, but you're lucky I'm working this case, Salaoui. Even though every single scrap of evidence points to you, I'm still looking elsewhere. Despite everything, I'm not entirely convinced of your guilt – so don't go and mess it up.'

Piroz had delivered those last words with a strange solemnity. As if he alone stood between me and the fate that awaited me.

A trap? Another trap? Piroz was clever.

'One last time, Salaoui, it's very important. Did you have both legs ten years ago?'

Piroz must have interpreted my silence as a pause for reflection, but I'd already made my decision.

I didn't believe him.

In his eyes, I was guilty. In the eyes of the other officers too. All the evidence, the witness testimony pointed in that direction.

What was my word worth against that?

Nothing.

I didn't know who they were, but they had set me up.

I had no choice, I had to escape the net that was tightening around me.

Now. Whatever the consequences.

The movement took less than a second. I leaned forward, just enough for my hands to grip the mahogany plinth of the model of the *Étoile-de-Noël* and, in the same movement, spun around with my arms raised to bring the plank of wood down on the head of the police captain.

Piroz didn't have time to react. He fell heavily to the ground. His hands clawed at the void while his legs no longer supported him. Only his eyes clung to me. Terrified.

A thread of blood slipped from his pleading mouth.

'Salaoui, no . . .'

No what?

What was he most afraid of losing?

His model? His prey? His life?

He tried to get back to his feet and rested both hands on the tiled floor. Dazed. Scarlet drops formed on his brow and dripped along his hair.

I glanced one last time at the *Étoile-de-Noël*, the fine rigging glued on with the precision of a watchmaker, the little sailors arranged in minute detail on the deck, then I smashed the whole thing against the back of Piroz's neck.

He fell to the ground, unconscious.

For a few minutes I stood frozen in place, sure that a dozen policemen alerted by the noise would suddenly appear in the office.

Silence. Closed door.

Almost as if they were used to people being beaten up within their walls.

I quickly assessed the situation. How was I going to get out of this now? Climb out the window? Sprint down the corridor to reception? Pull Piroz by the collar, with a letter opener pressed to his carotid artery, and make my escape by holding him in front of me?

Ridiculous!

My only hope was to leave as I had come in. Detached. Vaguely worried. A smile of complicity to the girl cop on reception.

As silently as possible I tugged on the apple-green cord of the shutter that was supposed to protect the room against the rare sunlight of Fécamp. It took me less than a minute to bind and gag Piroz.

He was breathing, but he wasn't moving. His eyes were closed, his eyelashes and hair sticky with blood. I took a few seconds to grab the green file in passing.

Magali Verron.

I thought of taking others. There was a great pile of files stacked up on the captain's desk, but I didn't have time to sort through them. I couldn't afford to weigh myself down either.

With one final movement I slipped into my pocket a loose page that was sticking out of the file. It was the one that had intrigued me the day before.

A simple table on a white background.

Eight numbers in four boxes.

2/2	3/0
0/3	1/1

One more mystery?

This one could wait . . .

I left.

A first policeman crossed my path; a second appeared on my right and brushed past me; two others came towards me at the end of the corridor, guns in their belts, stared at me, slowed down and stepped aside.

I passed between them without turning around.

I was already in the entrance hall.

'Did you survive?' the girl cop at reception joked.

I almost felt guilty for returning her smile. Her colleagues were going to blame her for what happened She had joked with the rapist on the run, never suspecting a thing, failing to raise the alarm. Would she dare to say that she'd thought he was nice? That he didn't fit the profile of a killer? That they were perhaps mistaken?

Given the lengths they'd gone to in their efforts to set me up, the ease with which I escaped seemed laughable.

As soon as I went down the steps of the police station, the iodine-filled wind lashed my face.

I was free.

For how long?

I quickly put some distance between myself and the station and headed towards the harbour.

How long before Piroz raised the alarm?

I thought fleetingly again of the five directions on my star. Becoming the one-legged hero of the Ultra-Trail of Mont Blanc, making love with the woman of my dreams, having a child, being mourned, paying my debt . . .

Not exactly a great start . . .

I would only escape the police for a few hours; a few days at most. I couldn't go back and sleep at the Sirène, or even head towards Yport.

What was I going to do?

Prove my innocence all by myself? Wait for this madness to evaporate like a bad dream? For the police to find another culprit? The real killer?

I left the seafront behind me. The place was deserted. In this weather, no one was venturing out. The pebbles on the beach swallowed me up without anyone noticing me.

Without anyone hearing me.

I'm innocent! I yelled in my head.

I'm innocent!

The water rose gently, but by walking quickly I was able to get far enough away before it covered the shoreline completely. Between Fécamp and Yport, over ten kilometres of shoreline, there was only one means of access to the sea, at Grainval, and dozens of panels indicated that it was strictly forbidden to walk below the cliffs.

The local police had long ago stopped playing hide-and-seek with the smugglers on the customs men's path. No one would come looking for me here, between sea and chalk.

The pebbles rolled beneath my feat. Already, Fécamp was just a vague line of grey buildings. Gripping the green file in my hands I thought again of Piroz and his accusations.

One question haunted me.

By hitting him and running away, had I torn free of the spider's web that was being woven around me?

Or had I taken one more step towards the abyss that was waiting to engulf me?

II
Arrest

Rosny-sous-Bois, 22 July 2014

From: M. Gérard Calmette, Director of the Disaster Victim Identification Unit (DVIU), Criminal Research Institute of the National Gendarmerie, Rosny-sous-Bois

To: Lieutenant Bertrand Donnadieu, National Gendarmerie, Territorial Brigade of the District of Étretat, Seine-Maritime

Dear Monsieur Donnadieu,

Following your letter of 13 July 2014, regarding the discovery of three skeletons on Yport beach on 12 July 2014, our service has devoted itself with utmost diligence to this troubling case.

Although to date none of the three individuals has been identified, preliminary forensic examinations confirm that the bones belong to three men, adults, aged between twenty and thirty at the time of their death.

We could find no evidence of significant trauma to the three skulls, or any other part of the skeletons, which seems to rule out the possibility that they were killed by the collapse of the cave walls. However, violent or non-natural death remains a possibility, taking into account the circumstances of the discovery of these bodies. Complementary chemical examinations will allow us to test the possibility of death by poisoning.

Establishing the time of death of these three individuals is proving to be one of the most disconcerting aspects of this inquiry. As is customary, we've given each of the three skeletons a temporary identifier that will

be used for the duration of the inquiry. In this case we have assigned three names whose alphabetical order corresponds to the chronology of their deaths.

In fact, and here we touch upon a particularly difficult point to explain, the three individuals died on three different dates, which rules out a death that we could term 'collective' or 'simultaneous', whether it was an accident that befell a group of cavers, a triple murder or indeed collective suicide.

The first of these skeletons, Albert, died no later than the summer of 2004.

The second, Bernard, died several months after Albert, probably between autumn 2004 and winter 2005.

The third, Clovis, died in 2014, between February and March, so about five months ago. Given the acidity of the chalk caves in which the corpses have lain since then, the swiftness of the decomposition of this last body seems hardly surprising.

To conclude, Lieutenant, and as you yourself observed in your letter, it seems difficult to dissociate the identification procedure of these three skeletons from the case commonly referred to as the 'red-scarf killer', one of whose victims, Morgane Avril, was found murdered in June 2004, not far from the place where the three skeletons were themselves discovered.

However, until we have the results of further examinations, including DNA analysis of the bones, we are unable to determine what direct connection there might be between the death of these three men about whom we know nothing and the murder of the girls.

Please rest assured, Lieutenant, that we doing everything in our power to progress this inquiry as speedily as possible. Unfortunately, as a result of recent cutbacks, our personnel cannot devote themselves to this case alone. Moreover, since the deaths of Albert and Bernard are covered by the ten-year statute of limitations, I regret to inform you that they cannot be considered a priority.

Cordial regards,
Gérard Calmette
Director, DVIU

18

How much longer?

For much of the afternoon I waited for night to fall, hiding in one of the countless caves in the cliff, a little way uphill from the Valleuse de Vaucotte, clinging like a mussel to the sections of rock face revealed by the swell.

Soaked.

A strip of pebbles about a metre wide was drying out between the sea and the chalk wall, but occasionally bolder waves amused themselves by crashing against the rock and drenching the idiot hiding there with their spray. By way of recompense for my efforts, a compassionate God had offered me the most sumptuous of sunsets, just before I climbed the reddening valley towards Vaucottes.

I waited again before leaving the trees of the Bois des Hogues. Ten minutes. Long enough for the darkness to become more intense, and for my wet clothes to stiffen into an icy shroud.

Still free, but deep frozen.

Grey night. In the gloom, the Valleuse de Vaucottes began to look like a haunted valley. The thirty or so houses lost in the jungle of pines, hazel trees and oaks, seem to have been built after a competition by architects who had been put under a curse. Each villa rivalled the next in baroque invention. Swiss chalet roofs, Tyrolian bell towers, English bow windows, Moorish façades. I checked that there were no cars about and then climbed up by the beach road. La Horsaine, the villa of Mona's thesis supervisor, was hidden just past the crossing.

Martin Denain,
123 Chemin du Couchant

'You'll find the keys under one of the bricks in the coping of the well,' Mona had told me on the phone. 'Near the cart. The gardener who looks after the grounds puts it back when he leaves. Make yourself at home. I'll join you as soon as I can.'

She had given me a virtual kiss and hung up. Without asking me any further questions, settling for the crazed account that I'd given her.

The cops are after me.

I need to hide.

You have to help me.

Mona was an amazing girl.

I found the iron key under the brick, the door opened, I took refuge behind the walls of La Horsaine.

Make yourself at home . . .

First a steaming shower. Then take stock. Tell Mona everything as soon as she gets there . . .

Before finding the bathroom, I wandered the maze of corridors, of tiny but innumerable rooms, staircases that connected three floors with plenty of half-landings. Apparently Martin Denain rarely came here. Not that the house wasn't well maintained – far from it. A gardener mowed the lawn and pruned the rose bushes impeccably, and a housekeeper must have been paid in gold to get rid of the colonies of spiders and polish the panes of all the windows on the top floor.

A clean villa . . . and an empty one.

It was this contrast that I noticed when I was contorting myself in front of the huge mirror, gilded with gold leaf, to slide my wet jeans along my leg. My prosthesis tapped against the blue Delft tiles. I had a sense that the echo was spreading through the thousand and one rooms of the deserted villa, waking shadows and ghosts.

The jet of water drowned out the noises of the house. I stood on one leg in the shower.

A flamingo-pink toilet! I was sure Mona would have liked the expression.

With my eyes closed, I imagined the interior decoration of La Horsaine. Martin Denain had stuffed the house, that was the right word. He had stuffed it. Flowers on the mantelpiece and the bed-heads. Artificial flowers. A basket of fruit on the kitchen table. Also artificial.

Shelves in the corridor with disorderly piles of paperbacks, magazines and games, which looked as if they had been forgotten there for decades.

As I let the hot water run over my naked skin, I reflected that this haunted-mansion décor seemed strange, almost unreal, as if drawn directly from the imagination of a novelist.

Like Mona's personality . . .

A scientific researcher who had appeared out of nowhere.

Lively. Pretty. Original and shameless.

As if she had sprung from the head of a writer . . . or mine, the head of a bachelor in search of love.

I raised my head to let the jet of water thump against my skin.

No, on reflection, the second hypothesis didn't stand up. Mona was insanely charming, but if I had to come up with a portrait of the ideal woman, she wasn't the one I would have drawn.

And as if by enchantment, under the cascade of hot water, it was the washed-out face of Magali Verron that danced in front of my eyes.

Make yourself at home . . .

I attached my prosthesis and grabbed a cream-coloured dressing gown hanging on a hook. A Calvin Klein. I thought of calling Mona. I had to be cautious, the police would be bound to make the connection between her and me. I knew she wouldn't blow my cover, but they might suspect her and follow her . . .

I banished those ideas from my head. I was still lost in the sequence of empty rooms, avoiding the reality that I had no strategy apart from running away. Not the slightest idea to prove my innocence, apart from gaining some time.

After half an hour I started finding my bearings in this baroque labyrinth. Apart from the basement, which was probably as huge as the villa itself, I had visited every room. In the drawing room, copper bottles were lined up on a cast-iron shelf.

Make yourself at home.

I poured myself a Calvados, a Boulard. The label said '*hors d'âge*'.
Ageless, like the house.

As soon as I had taken a sip, a fire raged in my throat. My coughing bounced off the walls and back into the silence, then drifted away in hiccups towards the upper floors, like a fearful poltergeist disturbed by an intruder. However much I scoured my memory, going back to my childhood in La Courneuve and the succession of flats from T0 to T5 that I had lived in as the family grew, never in my life had I set foot in such a massive dwelling.

It scared me a bit.

I chose to wait for Mona in the room that I'd dubbed the eagle's nest: it was the tallest room in the villa, built into a little tower that extended several metres beyond the roof and the chimney. From outside, I had seen that kitsch belfry for an architect's folly, a snobbish substitute for a castle keep. I was mistaken! In that circular eagle's nest, from every narrow window that looked like a romantic arrow slit, the view of the Valleuse de Vaucottes, the beach and the sea was stunning.

A lighthouse!

Martin Denain had put his office there. A library at a low level all the way around the edge of the room, encircling two Voltaire armchairs and an oak table covered with thick purple velvet.

I waited there for a long time, between the sky and the sea, perhaps more than an hour. My eyelids were starting to close when Mona's hands settled on my shoulders.

I hadn't heard her come in, hadn't heard her climb the stairs.

A fairy.

She was wearing the star of her wand over her heart.

'Thank you,' I said, even before I kissed her.

For a long time.

We stayed there for a moment, enjoying the moon and its quivering twin who was drowning in the Channel.

'Tell me,' Mona said at last.

I didn't hide anything from her. Piroz's accusations. My escape. My conviction. I was the victim of a police stitch-up. After listening to me, she interrupted me once. Mona uttered three words, the only ones I wanted to hear.

'I believe you.'

I kissed her again. I untied her golden hair and let it flood through my fingers.

'Why? Why are you doing this for me?'

Her hand slipped between the open flaps of my dressing gown.

'Have a guess? The scent of the unknown? An insatiable greed for unusual stories? An intimate conviction that you wouldn't hurt a fly . . .'

'Maybe not a fly. But a cop?'

She burst out laughing.

'If I tell you to call a lawyer and hand yourself over to the police tomorrow morning, will you do it?'

I held Mona tightly in my arms.

'No! I don't want to fall into their trap. I want to understand it for myself.'

'Understand what?'

'Everything! There must be a logical solution. A key to open the door out of this hall of mirrors.'

While Mona unearthed the treasures of the kitchen storeroom – foie gras, confit de canard and a red Bergerac – I opened the 'Magali Verron' file that I'd taken from Piroz's desk.

I swore inwardly: the file contained nothing that I didn't know already. Her detailed CV, which confirmed the information I had picked up on the internet, her childhood in Canada and then in the Val-de-Marne, the various schools she attended, her work for Bayer France. The other half of the file concerned her rape and murder. Complex medical reports listed each of her contusions, backed up by grim photographs, her blood group, her DNA, the details of her asphyxiation as the result of strangulation, which led to her death.

They were wrong, damn it all! By a few minutes, perhaps, but they were wrong.

I was sorry I hadn't taken more time to go through the files on Piroz's desk, to dig out the evidence on the Camus and Avril cases, clues other than the ones that some well-intentioned soul was drip-feeding me.

And also to find a clue to that series of figures Piroz was so interested in.

| 2/2 | 3/0 |
| 0/3 | 1/1 |

'Dinner is served!' Mona exclaimed, briefly dispelling the swarm of questions buzzing around in my head.

The thesis supervisor's larder was more than a match for the menu at the Sirène. Mona had merely placed the block of foie gras on the table and heated up the bits of confit in a bain-marie.

'To Martin!' she said, raising her glass of Bergerac. 'P@nshee pays him the equivalent of three trips around the world per year. We need to help him clear a bit of space at home.'

I clinked glasses, with a sad smile. My heart wasn't in it.

'What are you going to do?' Mona asked.

'I don't know.'

She spread the foie gras on a soft biscuit that she had found in a Tupperware container at the back of a cupboard.

'That's a shame. They're bound to catch you in the end. Then you'll lose everything. Everything I found charming about you.' Her finger caressed the star that she wore pinned to her blouse. 'That brilliant idea of hanging five dreams on your life. What . . . what are you going to do with those dreams?'

'I have no choice, Mona.'

She stared at me in silence for a long time, without taking the trouble to try and persuade me any further. The way you give up when faced with a stubborn child. Just as she was getting to her feet to pick up the saucepan behind her, the riff of my ringtone exploded into the room.

I picked it up.

'Salaoui?'

Piroz.

'Salaoui, don't hang up. Don't be an idiot. Hand yourself over, for fuck's sake. You will have the right to a lawyer. You will have access to the case file. You will be able to defend yourself.'

I decided to go on listening, for less than fifteen seconds, without saying a word. The bastard was doubtless trying to locate me.

'Salaoui, you've messed up badly, but we'll sort that out later. I've contacted the Saint Antoine Institute, all your colleagues, including the professionals, the psychotherapists. You're not alone! We can help you. Don't spoil your—'

Twenty-five seconds.

I hung up and turned my phone off, but my arm kept shaking. Gently, Mona rested her hand on mine. She was speaking even more gently than before, as if trying to tame me.

'In his own words, that cop was saying the same as me.'

Hand yourself in.

It would be so easy.

'They want to pin those murders on me, Mona. You heard him, with his shrinks and everything, they're going to say I'm insane . . .'

She gripped my hand even harder. I went on.

'My prints can't possibly be on that girl's body! I didn't touch her. The cops are lying. They're cooking something up. Why doesn't anyone know about Magali Verron's death?'

'I know about it, Jamal. André Jozwiak knows about it, and he must have passed on the news to all the locals who come to his bar.'

'It wasn't mentioned in the papers today.'

'It will be tomorrow . . . Jamal, why would the cops take the risk of inventing fake clues?'

'I don't know, Mona. But if you want to play at riddles, if you want to ask questions, I've got boxes full of them! Why is someone going to the trouble of sending me those envelopes that tell me

157

every detail of the Avril–Camus case? Why did Magali Verron take her life after copying Morgane Avril's life? Why was that red cashmere scarf hanging in my path like a beacon?'

Mona pushed the block of foie gras around in front of her, almost untouched.

'OK, you win. I'll hand myself in.'

With a pair of stainless-steel tongs she lifted out the two duck legs. Crimson. They made me think of two legs pulled from the body of a new-born baby that had been kept in a jar by a medical examiner. Even though I didn't bat an eyelid, Mona noticed my disgust. She put a hand on my shoulder.

'I know you're not a murderer! It hadn't even crossed my mind. But someone believes it . . .'

The boiled meat made me feel like throwing up.

'Why me, for Christ's sake?'

Mona took the time to think. I was touched by her expression of extreme concentration, her nostrils twitching, her eyelashes beating, her incisors biting her lower lip.

'Why you . . . That's the right question, Jamal. Have you ever been to Yport? Before this week?'

'No.'

Her teeth released her lip, ready to bite me.

'I want the truth, Jamal! I'm not a cop. If you want me to help you, stop playing games.'

'No,' I said. 'But . . . but nearly.'

'For Christ's sake, Jamal, tell me what happened.'

'It was about ten years ago. I was chatting on the net with a girl I liked, I'd got off with her one weekend by the sea, she was heading for Étretat, but it was too expensive for me, so I booked a room near the Needle. Here, in Yport.'

'And?'

'And, when she saw that her prince charming had only one leg, the cow called off our honeymoon.'

'You hadn't told her?'

'I'd forgotten to put a webcam under my desk . . .'

'OK. And you've never set foot in Yport?'

'Not even one!'

Mona laughed. She topped up our Bergerac.

'Sorry. I'll add your lousy date to the list of coincidences! And this week, what on earth brought you here? Wasn't there anywhere else to prepare for your limping run on the glaciers?'

'A few months ago I did a survey on the phone. Something about tourism in Normandy. There was a draw attached. I won a week in a hotel in Yport. Half board included, and all the ups and downs of the Paris Basin as my playground . . . You can see why I didn't have to think very long before burying myself away down here.'

'I get it.'

Mona drained her glass, walked to the window and then looked up at the tower whose shadow could be made out above the roof.

'We'll have to be sensible, Jamal, I'm not going to be able to sleep here. The police will quickly make the connection between you and me. They'll turn up at the Sirène with a warrant for your arrest tomorrow morning.'

I walked over and put my hand on her waist.

'We have time before tomorrow morning, don't we?'

Her eye slid to the dark hairs on my torso, which contrasted with the pale down of my open dressing gown.

'Not here,' she murmured, staring at the eagle's nest. 'Up there . . .'

19

The scent of the unknown?

Mona had decided to have a shower before joining me in the round room that dominated the villa. I heard her footsteps on the stairs. She too was wrapped in a Calvin Klein dressing gown. Ruby-coloured.

She kissed me on the lips, admired the panorama for a moment, the sleepy valley lapped by the blind waves, then she darted across the room to pick up a dog-eared old book from one of the shelves of the library. She jumped gracefully on to the purple leather desk.

'Maurice Leblanc!' she announced, flourishing the yellowing volume. 'The creator of Arsène Lupin. He wrote his first novels here, in Vaucottes. He even used the valley as the setting for one of his short stories . . .'

I wasn't listening to what she was saying.

I wanted to forget the Verron–Avril–Camus case.

I wanted to forget the cops on my heels.

I wanted to forget everything but Mona's white body in her ruby-coloured dressing gown.

She lifted one knee on to the desk so that the towelling fabric, held at the waist by a cotton belt, opened a few centimetres.

'Listen to me, Jamal, you'll be interested in this story by Maurice Leblanc. It's the story of some poor wretch who walks by one of the Vaucotte manor houses. His name is Linan – cute, don't you think? He comes in to steal something to feed his sickly children. But he's unlucky, because a few minutes before the owner of the mansion had fired a bullet into his head. A suicide!'

I walked over to her. I slowly parted the dressing gown to reveal her alabaster breasts.

'And then?'

A little flick. The dressing gown slipped gently over her naked skin, to her waist. Mona was now a red fruit whose peel had been removed the better to enjoy the flesh. She let my hands run over her breasts. Her voice faltered a little, but she didn't lose the thread of her story.

'Linan makes too much noise, he panics, knocks something over, the maid turns up, finds him at the foot of her master's body . . . You can guess the rest. Arrest. Trial. Everyone thinks that poor Linan killed the owner of the house, and no one believes the suicide story.'

My hands were moving lower now, to her belly, stopping at the ruby-coloured belt tied over her navel. I whispered in her ear.

'And how does it end?'

A shiver ran down the back of her neck. She raised the book level with her breasts.

'Hmmm. You want me to read you the last lines? Listen, it's educational, you'll love it.'

'*Justice rang at the door one day.*

'"*Prepare to die, Linan.*"

'*He was washed. His hands were tied. He allowed himself to be led like a docile animal, like an object. They had to carry him to the scaffold.*

'*His teeth chattered. He stammered.*

'"*I didn't kill nobody . . . I didn't kill nobody.*"'

Under the pressure of my fingers the belt of the dressing gown slipped around her waist. The two strips of red cotton opened like a rose at the first ray of sunlight.

'"The Scaffold",' Mona whispered. 'A short story published in *Gil Blas* on 6 February 1893. One of the first pamphlets against the death penalty!'

She set the book down and sat straight-backed on the desk. She reminded me of Madame Concetti, the English teacher who had inspired an entire class of fourth years. Although she had been dressed, at least.

My hands ran over her naked hips.

A suicide? An innocent. A nonsensical murder story pinned on him. Thank you, Mona. Message received.

'And you wanted me to hand myself in to the cops?'

I leaned against the desk. While I pressed my lips to her neck, by some magic trick, her foot untied the belt of my dressing gown. She didn't stop there, her toes set off exploring under the open folds of cream cotton.

Suddenly she laid both her hands flat on the purple desktop and arched her back. Her breasts pointed at the ceiling. Twin peaks born of a single eruption. I clung to them with both hands as my tongue ran down the slope of her belly, an interminable slide that left me intoxicated, leading to a moist meadow at the bottom.

Mona slept on the velvet desktop, curled up like a child. As she sank into sleep, she had made me promise to wake her before daybreak so that she could flee to her room in the Sirène.

A pretty little vampire . . . Sensual and enterprising.

I hadn't been able to stop myself wondering what excited Mona the most. Making love with a man on the run, accused of rape and murder, or abandoning herself to that man on the desk of her thesis supervisor, her body feverish, in the very spot where he must have written most of his work?

Both, probably.

I wasn't sleepy. I did a tour of the room, both literally and figuratively. For some hours my eyes had been lost among the stars lit by the outgoing tide, Mona's naked body and the hundreds of books surrounding me.

Old paperbacks rubbed shoulders with huge collections of photographs, thick scientific manuals and dozens of box files. I mechanically read the inscriptions on their edges.

1978–1983–1990–1998–2004.

2004?

The year of the murder of Morgane Avril and Myrtille Camus.

I walked over and opened the box. I expected to find printouts of lecture notes, students' essays, photocopies of research articles.

I was completely wrong.

I bit my lip to keep from crying out.

Professor Martin Denain, specialist in molecular chemistry, had amused himself by cutting out all the articles in the Courrier Cauchois *about the Morgane Avril case.*

I feverishly set the file down on the nearest chair and picked up some pieces of paper at random. The yellowed cuttings all told the same story, the one I had read in the documents sent to me by a stranger.

Nothing new, I was already familiar with most of the articles.

Nothing new . . . with one exception.

Why had this professor, who never set foot in Yport, collected these newspaper stories?

I thought of waking Mona to ask her the question.

Later.

I leaned over the box again, I had the whole of the rest of the night to read these articles, in search of a detail that might have escaped me and which might provide that spark, that famous key that would explain everything.

Naive as I was . . .

I had already been through about ten articles when I opened a colour double-page spread.

Avril case.

Special edition of the Courrier Cauchois.

Thursday, 17 June 2004.

'Of you, Morgane', was the title of the long article, a reference to a song by the singer Renaud.

I sat down to read it calmly.

I didn't immediately spot the huge photograph of the girl, smiling, in an oriental costume, probably at a *raqs sharqi* performance.

Then I stopped, arms dangling, mouth open. For the first time I saw Morgane Avril's face. None of the articles posted to me had contained photographs of her. Or someone had been careful to cut them out. Now I understood why.

I yelled like a madman.

The circular room around me vibrated like a rocket going off.

'Christ! It can't be her!'

My disbelieving eyes settled on the article again.

It wasn't Morgane Avril who had been captured in a full-page photograph in that newspaper from 2004 . . .

It was Magali Verron! The girl born ten years later who had thrown herself from the top of the cliff, in front of my eyes. Yesterday.

Mona woke with a start. She put on the dressing gown without even tying the belt and came anxiously over to me.

'A nightmare?'

Trembling, I held out the double-page spread.

'Bloody hell. Look at this photograph, Mona.'

She read the headline, 'Of you, Morgane', then concentrated on the picture.

'She was incredibly beautiful,' she murmured.

'Damn it . . . Mona, you're going to think I'm insane . . .'

'No, really?'

I ran my hand over her lips to erase her ironic smile.

'That girl in the photograph. The one they call Morgane Avril in this old newspaper. She's the one who committed suicide yesterday. It's . . . Magali Verron.'

Mona stared at me for a long time, as if her brain were trying to solve a complex equation, to assess all the parameters before formulating a hypothesis. She mechanically drew together the two sides of her dressing gown, which immediately fell open again.

'They look similar, Jamal.'

'No, Mona! It's not a simple resemblance. It's . . . Shit, it's her!'

'You only saw Magali for a few seconds . . .'

'Perhaps. But her face is engraved on my memory, you can understand that, can't you? Every tiny part of her face . . .'

'You talk as if you were in love with her.'

Mona had said those words calmly. A bit cynical. Rather than reply, I turned my back on her to search the rest of the box file. As I ran through the articles, I saw other photographs of Morgane Avril, full face, in profile, centred on her face or framing the whole of her body.

It was her! As ridiculous as it might have seemed, it was Magali, I was sure of it, I couldn't be mistaken.

Mona now seemed alarmed by my obsession. She pulled her dressing gown tightly around her neck, gripped the edge of the desk and stared at me as if I was a slow-witted student.

'Dear God, Jamal, think for two seconds. There are some incredibly shadowy areas in this case, we agree on that, but there are at least two absolute certainties. The first is that Morgane Avril died on 5 June 2004. All the national media led with that, all the police in France worked for months on this case. The second certainty is that Magali Verron died on 19 February 2014, yesterday, and you were an eye witness. I'm willing to go along with you on everything else, but those two deaths are axiomatic.'

'They're what?'

'Axiomatic! Facts that you can take as certain, on which you can base a reasoned argument.'

'Go on! What's your reasoned argument?'

Mona pointed to a photograph of Morgane Avril from *L'Éclaireur Baryon*.

'Well, we know that Magali Verron tried to be like Morgane Avril. Ten years later. Same schools, same tastes, same job . . . Same death. A crazy imitation. It's not so surprising, in the end, that she should also have tried to look like her physically.'

'She didn't just look like her, Mona. It's her!'

'So more than a physical resemblance? Is that what you're saying?'

Mona was on fire. I was starting to understand what it was that made her an excellent researcher: she was capable of finding a plausible explanation for any paradox.

'Even though they didn't know each other, Magali and Morgane may have been related! You told me that Morgane was born after a course of IVF, in Belgium? Magali might have been born to the same biological father, ten years later. She discovers the photograph of Morgane, perhaps when her murder is reported on television news bulletins. She wonders about that resemblance, she does some research, discovers that they have the same father, she's traumatised by that . . .'

'So much so that she simulates a rape and a strangling, then throws herself off a cliff?'

'Why not? I'm looking, Jamal. I'm looking for rational explanations, like you.'

'There's nothing rational in this case . . .'

A heavy silence settled in the room. We were two lighthouse keepers cut off by a storm from the rest of the world.

I said it again:

'Nothing rational. Why, for example, did your thesis supervisor, who never comes here, take the time to collect cuttings from a local newspaper?'

'In 2004, he was applying for accreditation as a director of studies, which involved writing a dissertation several hundred pages long, a compulsory stage in becoming a university professor. He had a grant from the National Centre for Scientific Research. A year without classes. He spent several months here, talking only to the pebbles, to his microscope and his word processor. I imagine he got bored. He must have been excited by this case which was happening only a few kilometres from his study. Like everyone in the area.'

Like everyone in the area.

Once again, Mona had thought of everything!

I had a sense that she was teaching me a lesson that she had learned by heart.

'Weird, isn't it? Every time a researcher comes to Yport to collect pebbles, a girl commits suicide!'

I regretted my reply even before I'd finished it. Mona didn't even bother to get up. She ruffled her hair, put Maurice Leblanc's book back on the shelf, then mechanically tied the dressing gown around her waist.

Calm. Natural.

'I'm going to get dressed, Jamal. It's three o'clock in the morning. I've got to go back to the Sirène. The cops are bound to interview me about last night, about the dinner we had together, our double room, our lie-in. I'm going to have to tell them that you were just a one-night stand, that I found you a bit paranoid, with those twisted stories of yours. And no, my God, no, I haven't the faintest idea where you get them from.'

'I trust you, Mona. You're very good at telling stories.'

It was all I could think of. My delirious imagination, which had charmed her before, had fled. I watched Mona going downstairs.

She turned to look at me one last time.

'Just one technical detail, Jamal. Our research group collects pebbles in Yport every year, and has done since our lab has been in existence – almost exactly twenty-three years.'

She disappeared. Leaving me alone as lighthouse keeper.

She thought I was mad. Who could blame her?

Through the window I watched Mona's Fiat 500 manoeuvring its way down the gravel driveway and disappearing around the first bend.

Obey her? Give up? Call the police? Wait for them to come and get me?

Not yet!

I hadn't used up all my options before laying down my weapons. I wasn't the only witness. Christian Le Medef and old Denise had also looked at the cold face of Magali Verron; they could compare it with the face of Morgane Avril.

No logic could shake my conviction.

It was more than a passing resemblance.

20

A nightmare?

It was just after four o'clock in the morning when I set off, torch in hand. I walked for two kilometres to Yport, along the sea, at the foot of the cliff.

I hadn't slept. I would have time tomorrow. All day, holed up in one of the basement rooms of my haunted manor house. Unless the cops were clever and discovered my hiding place. Unless Mona gave me away first.

In the light of my torch, the chalk wall looked like the battlements of a fortress, as impregnable as they were endless.

Yport slept. In the reflection of the blue neon of the casino that lit up the night, I looked around for Mona's Fiat among the ten or so cars parked in the car park on the seafront. I couldn't see it. Mona had probably left it in one of the nearby streets.

All of the pastel-coloured shutters of the rooms of the Sirène were closed.

Mine.

The one where Mona was sleeping. On her own.

An invisible hand gripped my heart. I forced myself to keep on going to the dark sea wall, without allowing my mind to wander any further. I couldn't waste any more time. The last two hundred metres I had to cover would be the riskiest, all kinds of danger might lurk concealed in the deserted street of the village. The police must have put a price on my head, or something of the kind, an appeal for information, a nice reward for anyone who could hand over the limping rapist. I had never felt so vulnerable. I couldn't just melt away into the labyrinth of stairways and underground car parks that linked the different tower blocks of the Cité des 4000 estate.

Two hundred metres in the open to get to Christian Le Medef's house.

I walked forward in silence, not disturbing the sleep of the Yport locals with a gloomy tap, tap, tap, like Long John Silver coming back to the *Hispaniola*. Over time, I had learned to slide the prosthesis of my left foot a few millimetres away from the tarmac.

A noise made me jump.

Behind me.

I sped up, then stopped abruptly.

The noise continued. It intensified. Came closer.

I pressed myself into the shadow of the coach gate of the estate agent's office, my heart pounding at one hundred beats an hour.

Rough breathing echoed down the cold street. The sound of footsteps on the pavement accelerated. Long seconds stretched out to infinity, then the shadow was on me.

The old dog looked as surprised as I was to come across a night-time stroller.

I put my finger to my lips to tell him not to make another sound. He sat down obediently, but then got up again as soon as I set off along the street again, always staying a few metres behind me.

His yellow eyes behind me looked like two headlights that had ceased to give off light. The poor night-grey dog walked on three legs. No wooden, aluminium or carbon paw to give him relief, just a stiff furry stump, drawn up at a right angle. Perhaps he was just following me out of jealousy?

I stopped in front of Le Medef's house. I immediately saw rays of light filtering from under the closed shutters of the first-floor room.

My witness wasn't sleeping! A depressive insomniac, I would have bet.

The dog sat down on the pavement opposite to wait for me.

I pushed the gate, then knocked gently on the door.

No reply.

I turned the handle, convinced that it wouldn't yield, and that I would have to find a way to alert Christian Le Medef to my visit without waking up the whole neighbourhood.

Not a bit!

The door opened as if Le Medef was waiting for my visit. I introduced one foot into the house and said in a low voice, almost a murmur:

'Christian? Christian Le Medef?'

I didn't want that paranoid loner to shoot at me.

'Le Medef? It's Salaoui . . .'

No reply. The light upstairs illuminated the top of the staircase. Le Medef was probably stuffed full of sleeping tablets.

Xanax . . .

As I climbed the stairs I made a point of bringing my foot down heavily on each step. The rickety banister shook under my damp hand, I even thought it was going to come away. Wasn't Christian Le Medef being paid to maintain this house?'

My foot caught on the carpet on the landing.

'Christian?'

Still no reaction.

I carefully pushed open the bedroom door, expecting to find Le Medef collapsed on the bed, drugged up or drunk.

My eyes gazed into the void.

There was no one in the room. The bed was made impeccably. There was a book on the bedside table, just beside the burning lamp. Some clothes, a pair of pyjamas, a T-shirt and a beige pullover folded on a stand.

A bachelor's room!

I stopped to think in silence. I was distracted by something that sounded like a crackling noise. I went back down the stairs four at a time.

A bachelor's room, I repeated in my head. But a bachelor who gets up early! Apparently Le Medef was up already. The humming sound that I could hear was a badly tuned transistor radio! Le Medef was probably having his breakfast. I stepped forward on the black-and-white tiles. Apart from the corridor, there was only one room on the ground floor, a kitchen that opened on to a little dining room.

A table in the centre. A chair.

I stayed in the doorway, silent and motionless.

Christ, what could have happened?

There was a plate on the table. A slice of overcooked meat floated in a seat of tagliatelle. A glass of red wine placed in front of it, half full. An almost empty bottle. A knife, a fork, a checked napkin balanced on the edge. A half-baguette.

No trace of Le Medef.

'Christian?' I called again.

'France Bleu, at the end of the night,' the transistor replied faintly, before playing 'Mon Vieux' by Daniel Guichard. I called out more loudly, just in case he was in the toilet or the shower.

To no avail.

Le Medef hadn't slept at home tonight.

He hadn't even finished last night's dinner.

My brain faltered.

Christ, what could have happened?

For the next few minutes, I searched every available corner of the cottage. Since it had barely sixty square metres of floor space, that didn't take long. The only certainty was that Le Medef wasn't hiding there. And neither was his corpse . . .

Nothing. Just a few of the unemployed man's personal belongings, some clothes, some books, a laptop for which I didn't have the password, an almost full fridge, local newspapers, a whole pile of them, medication, antidepressants; not Xanax: Anafranil.

As if Le Medef had had to leave in a hurry.

When?

Without worrying about leaving fingerprints, I touched the bread on the table. Soft.

171

I poked the ashes in the fireplace. Warm.

Le Medef had probably disappeared less than ten hours ago, probably at dinner time. That was more or less the time when Mona had joined me in Vaucottes. I glanced around the room once more. It reminded me of Uncle Youssef's apartment. I was seven years old when I went there with my mother. He had died of a heart attack three hours before, and my mother had to get some papers for the funeral. His cold soup was still in a bowl, along with a barely nibbled slice of bread and two slippers under the chair.

Was Christian Le Medef dead?

Had he been killed? Kidnapped? Forced out of his home?

Why?

His last words, uttered yesterday outside the newsagent's, echoed in my head.

I'm going to keep on digging, see what else I can find out about Magali Verron. It's not normal, this omertà.

Had he found something?

He believed in a plot, a stitch-up.

The silence of the newspapers.

The silence of the police.

Had they taken him away to keep him from talking?

'Ridiculous!' a sensible little voice whispered in my head. In France, the police don't take citizens away in the night, without even giving them time to finish their dinner.

I consulted my watch: 4.35. I gave myself another ten minutes to look around the house before setting off for Vaucottes again. Before Yport woke up. I opened the drawers, ran my hand under the furniture, took the books out of their shelves, the clothes from their wardrobe. Nothing.

Apart from one detail.

A white sheet of paper folded in the phone book, on which someone, probably Le Medef, had scribbled a series of numbers in four boxes.

2/2	3/0
0/3	1/1

My fingers trembled as I closed the Yellow Pages. Was Le Medef on the same trail as Piroz? Was that why he had been eliminated?

Droplets of sweat ran from my arms to my hands, drenching every object I touched.

Handles, latches, switches . . .

Litres of DNA that would let them pin the disappearance of Christian Le Medef on me as soon as the neighbours sounded the alert.

I glanced through the shutters. The street was still deserted apart from the three-legged dog under the street light.

I folded the piece of paper with the eight numbers on it, put it in my pocket and left.

21

Had he found something?

I slept until ten in the morning. It was a text from Mona that woke me.

Cops called at the Sirène.
Looking for you. Said nothing.
Want you alive I think. Phew!
Take care of yourself.
Bonnie

I stood there motionless for several long seconds. I savoured the moment. The rays of the sun hanging over the Valleuse de Vaucottes passed through the panes of glass to gild the linen sheets. I rolled the huge eiderdown under my back and tapped in a reply:

They'll never take me!
Mystery no. 123: Christian Le Medef, aka Xanax, witness no. 2 to Magali Verron's suicide, missing since last night.
A trap!
Be careful.
Clyde

I waited several moments for Mona's reply. Which never came.
Get up. Wash. Get dressed. Have breakfast. Calm down.
Mona must have been limiting our correspondence on purpose.

She was right. The cops had met her, they might suspect her. They might be keeping an eye on her.

At about eleven in the morning, after emptying a box of Lotus Speculoos biscuits dunked in coffee, I went down to the basement, the only place in Martin Denain's house that I hadn't yet explored.

The next stage in my battle plan was quite vague in my head. To hide out in this villa all day, and use the communication tools at my disposal in the hope of finding a trail. Internet. Telephone. Like that guy in the Hitchcock film who solves an investigation without leaving his apartment, with one leg in plaster.

Given the thick layer of dust, no one could have set foot in the professor's basement for months. My asymmetrical footsteps imprinted themselves on the grey concrete, more immediately recognisable than if I had been walking in snow. When the bare bulb hanging from its electric wire came on, a smell of grilled insect spread through the room.

A collection of cumbersome objects whose use was reserved for sunny weekends was piled up in front of me. Bicycles, a parasol, loungers, a barbecue, garden furniture, a badminton net, balls, racquets.

Cardboard boxes were stacked up against the walls.

I had a whole day ahead of me, so I got stuck in and pulled the brown tape from the first box in the pile. It contained a dozen photograph albums.

I flicked through them, taking my time, as if each volume corresponded to an episode from a sitcom.

The Denain Family, season 1.

The university professor was posing in front of the Étretat Needle, in the 1980s, judging by the orange Renault 5 parked behind them, hand in hand with his wife, a pretty, slender blonde with her hair loose, smiling. His life played out with the photographs, held in place under cellophane. Martin on the beach. Martin the handyman. Martin the fisherman.

Another album. Denain, older now, again posing in front of

the Étretat Needle, in the 2000s, judging by the Audi A4 parked behind them, hand in hand with his wife, a slightly stout blonde, short hair, a severe expression. Martin surfing. Martin golfing. Martin playing tennis with his son, a brown-haired boy who must have been my age, and whom we saw growing up with the passing pages, and with the sequence of his holidays in the family's second home.

I went on looking through albums, at random, until I found what I was looking for: a photograph of Mona. There were two among the hundreds of shots.

In the first, Martin Denain was collecting pebbles with Mona. In the second, the researcher was posing with Mona in front of the Étretat Needle. Their hands didn't touch, but Mona was prettier than ever.

Professor Denain was a lucky guy.

As if by telepathy, my telephone pinged at that very moment. Bonnie's reply!

Tough luck with Le Medef, old pal.
Everything staked on witness no. 3. old Denise.
Otherwise, next stop straitjacket!

I smiled, then felt for the two-page spread from the *Courrier Cauchois* in my pocket. Mona was right. Le Medef was out of the game, so only Denise could testify that Magali Verron's face was identical to Morgane Avril's. Only Denise could prove that I wasn't completely insane . . . except that all I knew about her was her first name and her age.

Denise. Seventy years old.

A specimen as rare as a fifty-year-old Nathalie or a thirty-year-old Stéphanie.

I wasn't going to call all the Denises I could find in the phone book. Or ask Piroz for her address . . .

I nervously tapped in a brief reply. Two simple words in the form of an SOS.

Denise who?

As if Mona could know. Le Medef had told me he hadn't seen Denise in Yport. She might have lived in a village somewhere in the area.

I carried on exploring the basement.

On one of the highest shelves I found a small red box. I managed to make out the letters that had almost faded away:

Winchester AM Munition

A box of cartridges!

No ammunition without weapons . . . Obviously the professor must have hidden a revolver somewhere in the basement, probably safe from the children.

I searched for a good quarter of an hour before finding what I was looking for, in a chest to hidden away behind a stepladder and a ping-pong table. First I cleared away piles of clothes. Designer items, tossed there as if they were rags. Out of fashion? Too small? Forgotten? Worn Vuitton gloves. A pink Eden Park polo shirt. An Armani T-shirt for a teenager. A cotton Vichy-check tie with a Burberry label.

I let the piece of fabric slip between my fingers, reflecting that everyone with a bit of cash must have accessories like this in their wardrobes. I wasn't about to let my imagination run away with me and assume I was rummaging through the basement of the red-scarf killer aka Martin Denain, professor of molecular chemistry.

The revolver was hidden under the clothes.

A King Cobra, according to the inscription on the black metal. New. At least I assumed so; it was the first time I'd held a gun in my hand.

The message echoed around the basement just as my finger was testing the sensitivity of the trigger.

Ask the dog!

It had taken me a few seconds to understand Mona's message.

The dog? What dog?

At first I imagined a message with a double meaning, then I remembered Arnold, Denise's shih-tzu.

The fourth witness?

Mona was making fun of me!

I was trying to come up with a witty reply, along the lines of: 'If you have time on the beach, ask the seagulls', when my thumb froze above my phone's keyboard.

The solution exploded in my head as if it had been perfectly obvious all along.

Mona wasn't making fun of me!

Her advice couldn't have been more explicit. *Ask the dog!* With a bit of nerve and a lot of luck, it might work.

I raced up from the basement four steps at a time, without taking the time to tidy up the mess I'd left behind me. There must be a telephone directory in this house; I walked around the room looking for it, opening all the drawers in all the pieces of furniture.

The crunch of tyres in the garden of the villa made me freeze, as if an iron hand had scraped all the thoughts out of my skull.

The cops?

I instinctively ducked below the window.

I clearly heard the sound of a door opening. Footsteps on gravel . . . I wasn't going to let them find me here, like an idiot. I got cautiously to my feet and peered through the pane.

The car was parked outside the front door. The man was walking confidently towards it.

Even though it seemed completely impossible, even though the police hadn't got there:

He had found me.

He took the time to light a cigarette, then he didn't wait for a second.

The postman walked to the letter box and slipped through a big brown envelope, then got back into his yellow Kangoo and continued on his round.

22

A double meaning?

Jamal Salaoui
c/o Martin Denain
La Horsaine
123 Chemin du Couchant
Vaucottes
76111 Vattetot-sur-Mer

Shaking, I reread the address.

Jamal Salaoui
c/o Martin Denain

The handwritten lines danced in front of my eyes.

Who could have known that I was hiding here?

No one! No one apart from the one who had provided me with this hiding place.

The only person who was helping me to escape the police.

The only person in the world who believed me.

Mona.

Had she been play-acting with me since the beginning, since we met at the police station?

I looked again at the valley through the window, and my eye fell to the beach. What connection could my pebble-picker have with the death of Magali Verron? With the deaths of Morgane Avril

179

and Myrtille Camus? It made no sense. Only Mona could have posted this letter, but by sending me here, to the house of her thesis supervisor, she was clearly putting pointing the finger at herself.

Once again I gave up trying to understand. Curiosity overwhelmed me; I guessed that this envelope contained additional details about the Avril–Camus case, details that hadn't been mentioned on the internet or in the press.

I was sitting in the most comfortable armchair in the drawing room, beside the unlit fire. My hands were still trembling as they tore open the envelope.

It contained two pages.

Record of the statement of Frédéric Saint-Michel.
Exhibits MC-47, MC-48, MC-49, MC-50.

Myrtille Camus case – Monday, 30 August 2004

Ellen Nilsson had asked Commander Bastinet to let her take a statement from Frédéric Saint-Michel, the fiancé of Myrtille Camus. The commander had agreed to the criminal psychologist's request. He had his hands full with stacks of files, Judge Paul-Hugo Lagarde's demands, the guerrilla war orchestrated, via her lawyer, by Carmen Avril, who refused to believe that the police were doing everything in their power to find her daughter's murderer. And to add to the pressure, Bastinet was living with the fear that another corpse might turn up.

During the morning's impromptu debriefing by the coffee machine, Bastinet had noticed that his wrinkled features and the bags under his eyes contrasted with the psychologist's smooth forehead and delicate cheekbones. 'Five thousand euros!' Béranger, his deputy, had chuckled under his breath. The standard rate for a facelift.

Well out of Bastinet's price range!

How had a girl so preoccupied with her appearance ended up in a profession that consisted in delving into other people's private lives?

'Monsieur Saint-Michel?' the criminal psychologist asked, 'is this a letter from Myrtille?'

'Yes. The last one I received from her. She sent it to me from the camp, a few days before she died.'

Frédéric Saint-Michel was standing beside Alina Masson. She confirmed his words with a nod. The combative energy of Myrtille Camus's best friend contrasted with the brooding melancholy of Saint-Michel's expression.

'You didn't send each other texts?' Ellen pressed him.

'That too. But . . .'

Frédéric Saint-Michel found it difficult to talk about his fiancée. His fingers were gripping a cigarette pack in the depths of his pocket, and his eyes were pleading for permission to smoke in the station.

Alina Masson picked up the thread.

'Myrtille was a romantic. She liked letters. Letters on paper, I mean. She liked writing. While the camp was on, we sometimes finished our meetings after midnight, and she still made the effort to write in her tent by torchlight.'

Each character trait of Myrtille's, drawn from the lips of her best friend, seemed to pierce Saint-Michel like an arrow. He wedged an unlit cigarette between his lips and put his head in his hands. Ellen observed him the way an entomologist observes a fly bumping against the walls of an upturned glass. Despite his promise, Commander Bastinet couldn't resist butting in.

'Would you read that letter to us.'

Ellen frowned – as far as she was capable, given her suspiciously smooth forehead – then softened her superior's words in that reassuring voice:

'Monsieur Saint-Michel, I know that this is an intimate letter, a poem, from what you've told us. Probably the last words written by Myrtille before her life was taken. But perhaps we will find a clue in those words . . .'

Frédéric Saint-Michel crushed the cigarette in the hollow of his palm before replying, 'We were supposed to be getting married.'

Off topic.

The criminal psychologist fluttered her long eyelashes. Too long. False.

'I know, Frédéric. We'd like to hear what she wrote to you.'

Saint-Michel took the sheet of paper from his pocket as if it weighed more than a stack of books. His lips moved, but no sound came from them.

Under the desk, Ellen Nilsson laid her fingers, their crimson nails a perfect match for her amaranth-red dress, on the commander's knee. Startled at first, he soon realised that she was urging him to be patient.

She advanced towards the witness, her wrist hidden beneath a tunnel of bracelets.

'It doesn't matter, Frédéric. Give me the letter.'

The sheet of paper slid on to the desk. The criminal psychologist read in a firm, clear voice.

Myrtille, 24 August 2004, Isigny-sur-Mer, 2.25 a.m.

My love

> *I will steal time's wings*
> *To keep it from flying*

> *I will steal the day's crutches*
> *To keep it from rising*

> *I will steal spring's jonquils*
> *To keep it from fading*

> *I will steal the cocoon's caterpillar*
> *To keep it from escaping*

> *I will put grilles on the universe*
> *To keep it from parting us*

> *I will dress our good fortune in rags*

To keep it from buying us

I will kill all the other girls
To keep them from loving you

I will ask life for a family
To keep us from getting bored

I will build a fortress around us
And I will defend it

M2O

Alina Masson twisted a Kleenex to wipe the corner of her eyes. Frédéric Saint-Michel put a new cigarette between his lips and bit it until he left a groove between the filter and the tobacco, his expression blank.

'It's a wonderful poem,' Ellen said.

It wasn't an empty compliment, she really believed it. Myrtille had a gift. A talent that had been squandered like a handwritten page that someone crumples into a ball before throwing it in the bin.

She had a keener understanding of the reactions of those whose lives had been touched by Myrtille's charisma, reactions that lay between rage and despair. She had invited Charles and Louise Camus to witness the statement, but Myrtille's parents had politely declined. They no longer wanted to share the memory of their daughter with police officers or judges. Myrtille was buried in Elbeuf at the Saint-Étienne cemetery, and they liked to go and collect their thoughts there every morning. Alone. Talking endlessly to the investigators about the smallest details of Myrtille's life, they felt as if they were scattering her memories as one might scatter ashes.

Bastinet said nothing. Disappointed. Not that he was insensitive to these poignant verses, but he saw nothing in the poem that might help him to identify the killer, no matter how many times he read it. He let his finger run over the page.

'What's this signature, M2O?'

'Marriage, 2 October,' Saint-Michel explained. 'It's the date we'd chosen for the ceremony. The church in Orival, the town hall in Elbeuf. The community centre for the dinner and the party.'

He decapitated his cigarette and spat the stub into the palm of his hand. Alina set her damp Kleenex on the table.

'Can this poem really help you?'

Bastinet gave a slight shake of the head, unable to restrain himself. He couldn't bring himself to tell her that it had been a waste of time. The thing that would have helped them was Myrtille's sky-blue Moleskine notebook, the journal she wrote in every day, which might have contained details about the days and hours leading up to her rape. The notebook that the murderer had taken.

Bastinet rose to his feet. He stared at Frédéric Saint-Michel and thought he was nothing like Chichin the guitarist. It was hard to see what the young women at the community centre, including the lovely Myrtille, saw in him.

Bastinet headed for the door, explaining that he had urgent matters to attend to, that he would leave Ellen to finish the interview on her own, that she had his full confidence.

To go on talking about poetry, he thought. To ask about Myrtille Camus's incongruously sexy outfit on the day she was murdered, about the date of the wedding. Compassion wasn't going to help them solve this case. Aside from feeling good about doing the right thing, there was nothing to be gained from taking an interest in the victim. The investigation needed to focus on the murderer. During the twenty minutes that had been taken up by the interview, three calls had come in from people claiming to have recognised the stranger with the Adidas cap who had been prowling around Myrtille Camus before her death. So far this week they'd had dozens of these calls. He would have to follow up on every single one of them, though he was convinced it was a waste of time. This was not how they were going to catch the rapist.

*

184

The brigadier in charge of Valognes police station called him three hours later. Bastinet was busy trying to arrange for posters to be displayed in every tourist information office in the region showing the photofit of the man with the Addidas cap, and his twin with the red Burberry scarf. The suspect lived in his parents' holiday home, so they needed to target resorts, but those responsible for tourism were unwilling to cooperate.

'Put your posters up wherever you like, Commander, but not right under the noses of the tourists.'

Tourists? In September?

'Léo? This is Larochelle, Valognes brigade.'

'Yeah.'

There was a long silence from the brigadier. Get a move on, man, Bastinet thought.

But Larochelle couldn't resist milking his moment of triumph. But he had Bastinet on the edge of his seat a moment later:

'They've got him!'

'Who?'

'Your guy with the Adidas cap. The one who was hanging around the Camus girl. They picked him up in Morsalines. Trust me, there's no question it's him. And I've got his name and address!'

23

His name and address?

I read and reread the poem.

Moved. Disturbed.

Once again I wondered what connection there might be between the Myrtille Camus case . . . and me.

How did all these details add up? How could the investigation into the red-scarf killer's second crime help me to solve the first one, the murder of Morgane Avril? And the suicide of Magali Verron, two days ago? How would it get me out of this mess I found myself in?

I was in no rush to find out the name of the guy identified by the cops in Valognes, number one suspect in the murder of Myrtille Camus. Whoever was sending these packages was going to let me know. It was part of his plan.

I got up and walked into the drawing room, analysing each verse of the poem.

Something in the back of my mind kept nagging at me.

What if this wasn't a trap? What if someone was sending me these letters so that I could find the solution? So that I could discover, ten years on, some clue that the cops had missed. The identity of the double murderer.

The poem was one more piece of the puzzle.

I went to the window. Outside, a man in a tie was walking towards the beach, telephone wedged against his ear, turning frequently.

I ran through the questions jumbled up in my head:

Why send me those envelopes? Two days ago, I'd never heard of the case – what made them think I would be capable of solving it?

Who but Mona could have known that I was hiding in Martin Denain's second home?

Where had Christian Le Medef gone? Had he been kidnapped? Killed?

What was the significance of that table – four boxes and eight numbers – that both Le Medef and Piroz were so interested in?

A blonde was making her way down the steep slope, accompanied by two children with a four-wheel bike and a scooter.

Though I had no answers for the first four questions, they at least seemed logical and rational. Unlike the six that came next, each more insane than the last.

How could the cops have found my prints on Magali Verron's body when I never touched her?

How did she manage to wrap that red scarf around her neck as she fell off the cliff?

Why hadn't the media reported the death of Magali Verron?

What could explain the surreal coincidences between Magali Verron and Morgane Avril? Birth, tastes, education . . . and their identical features?

Was it possible, as I now believed, that Morgane Avril hadn't died ten years ago, even though her murder had made headlines?

And the subsidiary question.

Was it conceivable that one single parameter could resolve an equation with ten unknowns?

I took another glance through the window. The last member of the family, a teenager dragging his feet on the tarmac, cut off from the world, headphones the size of ear muffs.

I was certain of only one thing: I couldn't solve this mystery on my own, simply through the power of my little grey cells, as happens in old films where the investigator solves the case without even leaving his armchair.

I needed to act, and my first act would be to discover the identity of the third witness.

Denise.

Mona was right: I just needed to ask the dog for her address . . .

I searched Martin Denain's drawing room until I found the phone book under a pile of old newspapers. I flicked through the Yellow Pages. There were only three vets within a twenty-kilometre radius. I started with the closest one, the Abbatiale clinic in Fécamp. A purring secretary answered the phone.

'Excuse me,' I miaowed. 'I'm calling on behalf of my grand-mother, Denise, about her dog Arnold.'

'Arnold,' the girl replied in her sugary voice. 'One moment . . .'

The rattle of a keyboard sounded in my ear.

'Arnold, an eleven-year-old shih-tzu. Is that the one?'

I almost screamed with joy!

'Yes! How . . . how can I put it? My grandmother isn't always on the ball these days. She forgets appointments and vaccinations. So I'm taking over, for Arnold as well as everything else.'

'I understand, just give me a minute, I'll check.'

I heard the keyboard rattling again, then her voice came back on the line.

'We sent your grandma a reminder six months ago. Arnold needs to pay us a visit before June for his vaccination.'

'I knew it! Gran's forgotten. Can you send that letter again?'

'To your address or hers?'

'My grandmother's would be better. I call in every week.'

The secretary loved that. Her voice turned to barley sugar.

'I'll send that out today.'

I hesitated, timing it so I would catch her at the very last minute, right as she was about to hang up.

'Wait! Which address did my grandmother give you? Now that I think about it, the previous letter may have gone astray – we had to move her to a bungalow a few months ago.'

A brief silence, no typing this time. I guessed that she was spin-ning the rolodex.

'Denise Joubain, Ancienne Gare, Route des Ifs, Tourville-les-Ifs. Is that the right address?'

'Perfect, mademoiselle.'

Mademoiselle.

She chuckled a syrupy thank you and then I hung up.

The 1:25000 map was spread out on the drawing-room table. The hamlet of Les Ifs was six kilometres from Yport, in the middle of the countryside. I spent a long time highlighting the wooded areas, the isolated paths, to find a route that would get me to Denise Joubain while minimising the likelihood of being seen by anyone who might tip off the police. Six kilometres, a long way for a one-legged man to travel through forests and fields without being spotted.

Trying to meet the old lady was risky, but was it any riskier than staying in this place all day?

I had one last ace to play.

Denise and Arnold.

And now was the moment to play it.

24

Is she losing her mind?

I had been following the abandoned railway line for several kilometres. The old Fécamp line, which once connected with the Rouen–Le Havre train, hadn't survived the decline of tourism on the Normandy coast. All that was left was a long scar through the boggy fields. About ten metres deep. Now partially reclaimed by hazels, oaks and elms.

The rhythm of my stride was dictated by the space between the sleepers, rendered slippery by a cold drizzle. Until Tourville I hadn't encountered anyone beyond a few seagulls spying on me, and a buzzard, motionless on a tree stump, which seemed to have been waiting for a train to pass since the Belle Époque.

When I reached the hamlet of Les Ifs, I climbed the embankment and found myself outside the address where Denise Joubain was supposed to live.

The former railway station, the old station master's house, pastel blue, with roughcast walls and a slate roof, topped by two chimneys with orange chimney pots. According to the station clock, time had stopped here one day long ago at 7.34. No one had seen fit to remove the enamel 'Railway Station' sign. I could imagine the waiting-room door opening to reveal elegant ladies in crinolines, moustachioed bankers in boaters and Parisians in sailor costumes for a day at the seaside.

The trains were waiting for them.

About ten carriages and three locomotives lined the abandoned railway track. A carriage from the Orient Express, a Pullman car, a Pacific Chapelon locomotive. All looking as if they had still been in use the day before.

The setting seemed surreal to me, even though, while preparing my itinerary, I had discovered that an association of retired railwaymen had set up their headquarters alongside the old station. They were restoring the rolling stock so that railways companies all over the world could offer them a second youth.

The drizzle was more intense now, which probably explained why no one was tinkering on-site today. I made my way to the door, unable to shake the conviction that nothing would go as planned.

That Denise wouldn't be at home.

That she too would have been silenced.

That . . .

Arnold's yapping exploded behind the window, then his black snout appeared, topped by a lace curtain. He slobbered on the pane, hysterical, for two long minutes before Denise Joubain opened the door.

She opened her eyes wide as she stared at me from head to toe, as if, in my purple WindWall, I was time traveller from another century.

'Can I help you?'

She hadn't recognised me. And yet I had been careful to wear the same clothes as I was wearing the first time I met her, two days previously.

'Jamal. Jamal Salaoui. You remember: the beach at Yport. Magali Verron, the girl who committed suicide?'

Still plumbing the depths of her memory, Denise ushered me in without asking any further questions. Arnold looked at me suspiciously for a long time, then went and lay down on a green cushion that matched his lime-coloured pullover.

The big room that served as hall, dining room and sitting room was prettily decorated, with exposed beams, cupboards and Normandy dressers, lace and dried flowers, but what drew my eye were the photographs hanging on the walls. Dozens of photographs of trains, captured in the most beautiful landscapes in the world. Vast snow-covered steppes, Andean mountainsides, endless dykes crossing the sea.

'My husband was a railwayman,' Denise explained. 'Jacques passed away over nine years ago.'

She turned towards a poster of the Orient Express crossing the Venice Lagoon.

'We took full advantage.'

I reached into my pocket for the article torn from the *Courrier Cauchois* dated Thursday, 17 June 2004.

'Denise, I'd like to show you a photograph too.'

I held up the portrait of Morgane Avril, taking care to hide the headline and the date of the article. Even though the old woman was losing her memory, she couldn't have forgotten the face of Magali Verron after her suicide on the beach, two days earlier. The same face as the one in the newspaper.

'Do you recognise her?'

Denise excused herself and left me on my own for a few seconds while she went to fetch her glasses from the bedroom, the first door on our right. As I watched her walk way, it struck me that she seemed less alert than she had on Yport beach on the morning of the suicide. As if she had aged two years in two days. Finally she leaned over the photograph.

'Yes . . . that's the girl who died after being raped.'

It was all I could do not to hug her. As I had anticipated, she had confused the photograph of Morgane Avril with the face of Magali Verron. I wasn't going mad. I hadn't invented that incredible resemblance! Might this old lady become my ally?

I unfolded the article.

'Look at the date, Denise.'

She adjusted her glasses as if the clarity of her vision needed adjusting to the nearest millimetre.

'Thursday, 17 June 2004? My goodness . . . That terrible business seemed so recent . . .'

On the opposite wall, the Shinkansen was making its way between the skyscrapers of a Japanese city, perhaps Osaka.

'Two days?' I suggested.

Denise gave a tinkly laugh. She settled herself on a wooden chair with a wicker seat. Arnold took three leaps and landed on her knees. With a hint of irony in her voice, she told me:

'I know I'm losing my sense of time a little. But two days seems a bit much, doesn't it? But now that I think about it, the newspaper's right. Jacques was still alive when it all happened. He left me in 2005 . . .'

She raised a wrinkled hand, gesturing to me to take a seat. She still hadn't asked who I was or why I was asking her these questions. I took a chair and sat down facing her. Arnold sniffed me as if he was seriously thinking of switching knees.

It was all I could do to hide my excitement.

Denise remembered the murder of Morgane Avril!

It made sense, because she had been living here when it happened. But she didn't seem to have made the connection between the two girls who had died ten years apart.

'You're right,' I said. 'This is the photograph of Morgane Avril, the girl who was raped and murdered in Yport in 2004. But I came here to talk to you about the other girl, Magali – the one who killed herself the day before yesterday by jumping off the cliff.'

Her trembling hand ventured through Arnold's long fur. She looked at me as if she hadn't understood, as if she was about to ask me to repeat it, and then slowly uttered eight words:

'I was there when the corpse was found.'

Of course, Denise. So was I. We were both there. All three of us, if you count Le Medef.

She closed her eyes. I wondered if she had fallen asleep. She spoke slowly, as if describing a dream:

'I was walking on the beach. It was very early, I think, but it wasn't all that cold.' Her hand rubbed the belly of the shih-tzu, who groaned with pleasure. 'Arnold was very young at the time . . .'

An alarm went off somewhere in my brain.

Arnold? Very young?

'It was quite a strange day in Yport,' Denise continued. 'Young people were dancing all over the place outside the casino. There was

193

music, all night, rock music. I used to dance to rock music when I was their age, although a different kind, not the sort they were playing that evening. And it's strange, don't you think, that young people have changed their music but given it the same name? They all looked very happy. Before the tragedy, of course. Before they found the body of that poor girl at the bottom of the cliff.'

I fought the urge to grab that hairy bundle off Denise's lap and hurl it at the ceiling – anything to shock her brain into focusing on what happened two days ago, not ten years ago. I wanted to hear her confirm that I had never touched the corpse of Magali Verron.

Arnold pricked up his ears as I raised my voice:

'Madame Joubain, I didn't come here for you to talk to me about Morgane Avril, but about what happened when we met on Wednesday, two days go. You remember, when you went for walkies with Arnold on the beach at Yport.'

A smile brightened Denise's face. Arnold's tail began wagging at the word 'walkies'.

'My goodness, that's true, I had gone for a walk . . . So had Arnold. But it was so long ago. I don't go out very much these days, you know. And besides, Arnold's paws . . .'

What was this mad old cow on about?

So long ago . . . She was walking on the beach at Yport with Arnold only the day before yesterday!

Denise went on, as if unable to stem the tide of nostalgia.

'I'm like those abandoned trains out there. Like this rusty railway line. I sit here waiting and remembering. Every now and again a taxi comes to take me to the doctor, or to take Arnold to the vet. The home care lady even brings me my shopping.'

I stared at the frames on the wall. The trains were spinning before my eyes now. Denise followed the direction of my gaze.

'Jacques and I used to travel the world. It didn't cost us a penny. He was a brilliant engineer . . . In March 1962, the Baikal-Amur Magistral got stuck in snow just past Tayshet and—'

'I saw you at the police station, the day before yesterday,' I cut in. Arnold pricked his ears and bared his teeth, which were the size of melon pips. 'You were coming out of Captain Piroz's office.'

'Are you a police officer?' Denise stammered.

'No. No, quite the opposite.'

I immediately regretted saying 'quite the opposite'. At the risk of being bitten by Arnold, I rested a hand on Denise's knee.

'Are you frightened? Have you been asked to forget the incident the day before yesterday? Not to talk to anyone about it? Especially journalists?'

Denise leapt to her feet. Arnold squealed as he slipped down her legs.

'Are you a journalist? Is that it? You've come to dig up that old story?'

I got up too. Her wrinkled face was level with my neck. I was almost shouting:

'We spent over a quarter of an hour on the beach together, waiting for the police to arrive. You covered the body of that girl with my jacket. The girl had a red scarf around her neck . . .'

Denise took a few steps backwards. Hanging on a coat stand near the door I could see a grey raincoat, a straw hat and a beige silk scarf. Our eyes froze on that bit of fabric, then met.

I read the terror in Denise's eyes.

My hands settled on her shoulders as my voice became more gentle.

'I don't mean you any harm. I don't want to alarm you. All I want . . .'

At first I didn't understand what was going on. She rested her right hand on her left wrist, in a movement that seemed perfectly natural.

Then a loud beep exploded in the room as a red warning light blinked on her wrist, on her watch.

What I had assumed was a watch . . .

Denise, like a lot of old people who live alone, wore an alarm bracelet, presumably connected to her doctor's phone or the emergency services.

Damn it . . .

The paramedics would be here in a few minutes if she didn't deactivate that thing.

The phone rang a second later. She took a step to go and answer it, but I held her back by her sleeve. As soon as the answering machine clicked on, a worried voice rang out.

'Madame Joubain? Dr Charrier here. Is something wrong? Please pick up, Madame Joubain, is something wrong?'

The doctor was going to raise the alarm.

I had to get out of there . . .

I tried my luck. One last time.

'Denise, I beg you, look at me. Surely you recognise me?'

Her eyes passed through me as if I were a ghost, and the only interesting thing about me was the door I was standing in front of. Then, reassured by the imminent arrival of an ambulance, she replied in a calmer voice:

'Yes, I recognise you. You were near me, on the beach . . .'

Before I had time to savour that last hope, the old woman took my hand.

'You were younger too. Unlike the other boys, you weren't dancing. You could have done. You had both your legs in those days . . . You . . .'

I couldn't hear another word. I dashed outside, leaving the door open. The last image I had of the old railway station was Arnold running three metres into the car park and then barking as if to tell me never to set foot here again.

I darted through the gap between two carriages on breeze blocks, and ran to the abandoned railway line that stretched into infinity like a huge zip fastener a giant had closed over secrets buried underground.

'Hello, Mona?'

For the first time, I had decided to lie to her. At least by omission. I wasn't goiong to tell her that old Denise Joubain couldn't remember the accident two days ago . . . but that she had a perfect memory of the murder of Morgane Avril ten years before.

That she muddled everything, including the day when she had met me.

That she thought I was someone else.

That she was, quite simply, mad.

The phone rang out. The sleepers passed beneath my feet like an endless ladder to hell. In a hundred metres or so I would have to leave the abandoned railway to venture among the sloping fields of the Pays de Caux. The drizzle had turned into a cold fog that froze my skin, but at least it meant that if there were any hikers about in this weather, all they would see of me was a vague silhouette.

I was alone.

Christian Le Medef had disappeared. Denise Joubain was mad.

I was the only witness to the death of Magali Verron.

I nervously gripped my phone in my hand.

The only witness, apart from the cops. Apart from Piroz, his deputy and all the officers from the Fécamp brigade who had bent over that corpse.

No reply. Try again.

I pressed the green button on my iPhone.

'Hello, Mona?'

She picked up.

'So? Did you find your old woman?'

'No. Or rather yes, but it's complicated . . .'

'Tell me!'

'Later, Mona.'

I stopped under a hazel tree. Thick cold drops fell from the branches and then exploded on the synthetic fabric of my jacket.

'Can I borrow your car?'

For a few moments all I could hear at the other end was the sound of pebbles rolled by the sea, then Mona's playful voice asked,

'To hand yourself over to the cops?'

'No, Mona. To go Neufchâtel.'

'What?'

'To Neufchâtel-en-Bray. Carmen Avril, Morgane's mother, still runs her holiday home there, the Dos-d'Âne. It's less than an hour's drive away. I need check all the details. Mona . . . I need proof, I need you to . . .'

'OK, big man. Don't get overheated. Take my car if you

197

like. It isn't going anywhere, it's parked on the sea wall by the casino . . .'

I didn't even try to put into words the gratitude that I felt for Mona.

'By the casino? Damn! There's no way I can go anywhere near Yport beach in broad daylight, even in this weather. They'd nab me straight away . . .'

Mona sighed like a mother who has no choice but to yield to her little boy's whim.

'You're a pain, Jamal! I'll leave my Fiat by the road out of Yport, past the campsite, near the tennis courts. I'll leave the ignition key inside. The door and the boot haven't closed properly in years . . .'

'Thanks, Mona. I'll prove to you that you're backing the right—'

'Shut up! Hang up before I change my mind . . .'

Stuffing the phone into my pocket, I thought again of the postman, the brown envelope, my name on it, Martin Denain's address. An address that only Mona knew, Mona, to whom I had neglected to confess that there wasn't a single witness who could confirm my version of events . . .

Which of us was betraying the other?

I set off again along my icy path. The fog was getting thicker. I couldn't distinguish between the rows of poplars dividing the fields and the electricity pylons leading to the nuclear plant.

My testimony against everyone else's.

Who would believe me now?

Who would believe in my innocence?

No one . . .

No one but you?

At this point of no return into the depths of madness, are you still willing to believe what I've been telling you since the beginning?

I'm not making any of this up.

*

Are you still willing to back me?

I'm of sound mind. I haven't raped or killed anyone.

And I'm going to prove it.

25

Is something wrong?

The Fiat 500 sped at 130 kilometres an hour along the A13. My foot had been pressing the pedal to the floor for twenty kilometres so that I wouldn't lose speed as the road climbed gently towards the Pays de Bray.

I regularly checked that no one was following me, though there was really no need: the motorway was deserted apart from the occasional articulated lorry that appeared and then disappeared in my rear-view mirror. There was more traffic coming in the opposite direction. British drivers heading south, scrupulously respecting the speed limit, with skis and suitcases on the roof. Far from certain that they would get to the mountains before the snow had melted. Intermittent rain kept the wipers squeaking their complaints as they spread the scattered drops across the windscreen rather than wiping them away.

The monotonous plateau of the Pays de Caux suddenly gave way to a landscape made up of a patchwork of hedges. The motorway, after the long climb, toppled abruptly into the void before climbing up the slope on the other side. It was the first time I'd set eyes on the Pays de Bray, a kind of broad clay valley dug in the chalky plateau. Almost immediately I turned left in the direction of Neufchâtel-en-Bray.

The new houses seemed to have sprouted up along the interchange like mushrooms on a log. There were no tollbooths on the motorway, and Rouen was fifteen kilometres away. The sprawl of suburban housing had devoured the countryside for miles around.

The Fiat's thermometer indicated a temperature of 3 °C. In the middle of the afternoon, I had expected to enter a ghost town populated by a few old people braving the cold and the icy pavement between one shop and the next.

As soon as I'd crossed the bridge over the Arques, the anarchy of double-parked cars almost forced me to slam on the brakes.

What on earth were they all doing here?

A moment later, hordes of children in multicoloured caps began swarming through the maze of cars.

Four thirty. The end of the school day!

I turned at the first intersection to avoid the crowds. After weaving through a labyrinth of streets, between no-entry signs and dead ends, I parked in a deserted alleyway. I pulled my Nike cap low over my face, tugged my trousers down far enough to hide my prosthesis, then got out of the Fiat 500. The pavement was covered with revolting slush, in which my stiff leg drew a thin channel.

I plunged into the first available shop, its windows misted over.

I was betting that Piroz hadn't alerted every station in the region, and that the police wouldn't yet have managed to display my portrait in all the shop windows.

A greengrocer. The shopkeeper was busy building a pyramid of apples.

Organic fruit and vegetables, it said on a sign above the till.

'Can I help you?'

'I'm looking for a gîte – the Dos-d'Âne. Is it still run by Carmen Avril?'

The shopkeeper straightened. He was almost bald, apart from a tuft of hair that stood up like the leaves on a pineapple.

'What do you want from her?'

I tried to allay his suspicion with a forced smile.

'I'm a journalist, researching an article about the murder of her daughter, Morgane.'

Pineapple Stalk looked me up and down, much the same way his customers would examine a piece of fruit to see if it was ripe. I'd be fine as long as he didn't squeeze my leg.

'I don't think she'll be too happy about people troubling her with that kind of thing today. That's all in the past.'

'Ten years, to be precise,' I said. 'They want to reopen the case, a few months before the statute of limitation runs out.'

Without bothering to reply, he turned towards a display of berries. In the middle of winter, this idiot was selling organic strawberries, organic raspberries, organic cherries . . .

The sound of footsteps behind me made me start. A red-faced girl was carrying three boxes of red, white and green cabbages. Panting, she pushed past me unceremoniously.

'Carmen won't mind. She's not crazy about journalists, but even after all this time she'll talk to anyone who might help her catch the bastard who killed her daughter.'

Pineapple Stalk shrugged and grunted in his corner.

'They'll make us look like a village of weirdos.'

The girl arranged the three boxes on the floor in a staggered row.

'You'll find the Dos-d'Âne a kilometre beyond Neufchâtel, on the Foucarmont road. You can't miss the Gîtes de France sign.'

Just as I was leaving the shop she added, like a threat, 'Whatever you do, don't try and sweet-talk the woman.'

Some children were walking ahead of me as I returned to my car. Three abreast on the road to avoid the potholes in the pavement, which had turned into icy puddles. I didn't see a single parent accompanying them; perhaps they only picked up their children when the weather was fine.

That suited me. Fewer witnesses.

I blew on my cold fingers and opened the door of the Fiat.

My hand paused on the metal handle, as if frozen there.

There was a brown envelope on the passenger seat.

For Jamal Salaoui.

That handwriting, so familiar to me now.

Mona. She was the only one who knew I was going to Neufchâtel . . . but it was impossible for her to be here! How could she have got hold of another car? How could she have got to Bray before me, when I'd been driving with my foot down all the way? How could she have followed me when I'd spent half the journey staring into the rear-view mirror?

Why would she play such a sadistic game?

I sat down in the driver's seat. I turned on the ignition and put my hands against the vent to warm them up.

Who could have known that I was parked here?

No one.

Who could have slipped the envelope on to the seat?

Anyone. The car door didn't shut . . .

I waited for several long minutes, turning the heater up as far as it would go and aiming the vent at my face, until the hot air burned my skin. Then I opened the envelope.

Myrtille Camus case – Friday, 8 October 2004

Commander Léo Bastinet was reading the fax from Brigadier Larochelle for the third time, taking in every detail.

The stranger in the Adidas cap, number one suspect in the murder of Myrtille Camus, was called Olivier Roy.

He was twenty-one, he lived in Morsalines with his parents, who ran the newsagent's in Valogne. He was taking a course in cultural mediation at Caen.

Brigadier Larochelle had no right to claim credit for identifying the boy in the photofit. His parents, Monique and Gildas Roy, had presented themselves at the station in Valognes on 7 October 2004 to report the disappearance of their son. There was no doubt Olivier was the one the police were after. He had camped in Isigny-sur-Mer, sailed near the Îles Saint-Marcouf, and sunbathed on the beach at Grandcamp-Maisy on the dates when Myrtille Camus was there.

His parents explained that the murder of Myrtille Camus had affected Olivier, although they didn't really know why. As soon as the girl's death was reported in the press he had locked himself in his room for hours, only emerging for long solitary walks. On 6 October 2004, in the late afternoon, he had set off due north, along Boulevard des Dunes, towards Saint-Vaast-la-Hougue. He never came back.

For exactly thirty-seven hours Commander Bastinet thought they had their culprit. Olivier Roy's silence could have been interpreted as a desire to evade the police, his depression as remorse, his flight as a confession.

The next day, at around six in the evening, his suspicions collapsed like a house of cards.

Olivier Roy's DNA was not a match for the rapist's!

An hour later, a second piece of information dropped like a bomb: Olivier Roy couldn't have murdered Morgane Avril, nor could he have been the stranger with the red scarf described by Riff on the Cliff festival-goers. On the weekend of 5 June 2004, he had been at the street arts festival in Biarritz, nine hundred kilometres away, with three friends from his course.

The appearance and disappearance of Olivier Roy blew Bastinet's file apart. They pursued their line of inquiry for another few weeks. They took down the blurred photofit pictures and replaced them with the photograph of Olivier Roy.

But what was the point? Why bother trying to find someone who, at best, was merely a witness?

Judge Paul-Hugo Lagarde began to publicly question Bastinet's methods, while privately trying to get himself taken off this case before it scuppered his career. The local papers moved on, seizing upon the story of a worker from Mondeville who had asphyxiated himself with carbon dioxide, claiming the lives of his wife and four children who were in the car with him.

Criminal psychologist Ellen Nilsson took the Paris–Caen train less and less often, then not at all. The local police, who had been betting on which part of her body she would rejuvenate next through the miracle of Botox, had to find something else to bet on.

Everyone who had worked day and night on the investigation during the weeks following the murder of Myrtille Camus, had been driven by one fear: the discovery of a new victim. That fear had kept them at it, running a race against time, fuelled by adrenaline. Now they found themselves hoping that another rape would revive the case. They hoped in vain. The red-scarf killer had retired . . .

Carmen Avril met Léo Bastinet at the regional crime squad in Caen on 12 October 2004, a few days after the Olivier Roy trail was abandoned. She set down a heavy file on the commander's desk and proceeded to summarise what he would find inside.

The only way to discover the identity of Morgane and Myrtille's killer would be to look for someone who had been in Yport on 5 June 2004 and Isigny-sur-Mer on 26 August 2004. The likelihood of that person being innocent was almost nil, particularly since they had not voluntarily presented themselves to the police.

Bastinet nodded, and wearily opened the file. Inside he found lists, series of addresses, phone numbers, screenshots. Looking for a man, the commander thought, a man on his own, on the Normandy coast, first on one Saturday in spring and then one Thursday in late summer, meant having to check the names of every tourist who had booked into a campsite, a hotel room, a holiday cottage . . . And then there were the ones who had stayed with friends and family. The day-trippers who had used their bank card to pay a motorway toll, a restaurant bill, buy a souvenir in a shop. The ones who had left a business card or a cheque. Their face in a photograph.

The commander closed the file, then raised hollow eyes to Carmen.

'Madame Avril, I'm going to be frank. The budget for the Avril–Camus case has been reduced by ninety per cent. From fifty investigators we have dropped to five. In a few weeks, unless new evidence comes to light, not a single officer will be devoted exclusively to this case.'

Carmen Avril didn't bat an eyelid. Bastinet continued:

'Officially, since last week, this case isn't supposed to take up more than ten per cent of my time.'

He pushed the file towards her, without offering an assessment of the value of the work she had undertaken.

'We're not giving up, Madame Avril, but the investigation is on standby. We have the rapist's DNA, we know that he has claimed two victims. We have to wait . . .'

Bastinet was waiting for Carmen to dive in with a stinging retort: *Wait for what? Wait for him to rape another girl?*

He was disappointed.

Carmen gave herself a shake, tucked the file under her arm and marched out the door, yelling so that everyone on the floor could hear:

'We'll get by without you!'

In June 2004, after the murder of Morgane, Carmen had set up a collective. Everyone who had known Morgane had joined, almost five hundred people, but a hard core of about ten close friends had proved sufficiently active and, more importantly, sufficiently generous to help pay the fees of the lawyers in charge of the case.

The same evening Myrtille Camus's body was discovered, Carmen had invited Charles and Louise to join the collective. The next day they founded the Fil Rouge Association. The first article of the statutes consisted of two words:

Never forget.

Charles Camus became the association's president; his tact and diplomacy seemed more useful when it came to negotiating with the police and the legal system than the passion of Carmen Avril, who settled for the role of vice president. Carmen had always struggled in her dealings with men. Particularly men in authority. Océane, Morgane's sister, took care of admin. Alina Masson, Myrtille's best friend, was appointed treasurer. Assembling their dossier on the stranger who had been in both locations brought the two families together during the weeks after the second murder, but as soon as it was clear that no one would help them, the group splintered.

'We'll get by without you,' Morgane's mother had snapped at Commander Bastinet.

Carmen Avril was thinking crusade, vengeance, punishment.

Charles Camus was thinking truth, justice and even forgiveness.

*

The slender consensus within the Fil Rouge Association evaporated in 2005. Carmen had given her consent to a journalist from France 2 who wanted to devote an episode of *Bring in the Accused* to the red-scarf double murder. Charles had tried veto it, but Morgane's mother had argued that the TV broadcast would reach a huge number of potential witnesses, and the fee for their participation would help pay lawyers and investigators. The rest of the Avril clan lined up behind her. Louise Camus said nothing. Alina Masson and Frédéric Saint-Michel were initially reluctant to go against Charles, but in the end followed Carmen.

The programme was scheduled for 24 March 2005, at 10.30 p.m.

Like the other members of the Fil Rouge, Carmen first saw the ninety-minute programme at a preview screening held within the studios in La Plaine-Saint-Denis. The documentary traced the sequence of events and the twists and turns of the investigation, alternating murky reconstructions, indecent photographs of the victims and sorrowful testimony from neighbours. Without shedding the slightest bit of light on the case.

In the front row of the screening room, faces were expressionless.

Pure voyeurism! The double rape of Morgane and Myrtille had only been put on screen to compete with *CSI* or *NCIS* on the other channels. Carmen Avril wanted the broadcast to be cancelled, but France 2 held their ground. The show brought in an audience share of 18.6 per cent, which was slightly below average. The channel didn't pay a cent to the Fil Rouge Association, much less, posthumously, to its two leading actresses.

A few days later, Charles and Louise Camus announced their intention to distance themselves from the group. Charles, with customary diplomacy, cited a health problem as his reason for stepping down.

The last time they spoke to Carmen Avril was the day before the tragedy.

27 December 2007.

26

Wait for what? Wait for him to rape another girl?

I put the sheets back in the envelope and slipped it into the glove compartment of the Fiat 500.

So the two cases, of Morgane Avril and Myrtille Camus, had become one.

And within a year the case had been closed.

As I started the Fiat, I couldn't help smiling. This latest information would be useful to me.

Carmen Avril would welcome me with open arms. I had come to tell her that, ten years on, her daughter's murderer had emerged from his lair.

A few minutes later, I parked the car a hundred metres past the Gîtes de France sign. A woman was walking along the embankment, bent under the weight of three satchels. She was pulling a string of three children towards a cluster of new houses.

'I'm looking for Carmen Avril.'

The weary woman puffed.

'Down that driveway. You can't miss it. Hang on, there she is, out on her terrace.'

She pointed to a blue silhouette among the branches of the pollarded trees, then set off like a locomotive, towing her children behind her.

I set off down the driveway. The Dos-d'Âne was an old longhouse. The dressed stones of the building were in perfect harmony with the grey of winter, but it looked as though they would be covered in spring by wisteria or the blossom-covered branches of the big apple tree that stood in the middle of the courtyard.

On the terrace a stout woman armed with a hammer was busy straightening the screw bar of what I took to be an old apple press. A collector's item, which seemed to be in its rightful place in this garden which resembled a museum of Normandy's arts and crafts.

Carmen hammered away with force, energy and precision.

From behind, she looked like a man.

Suddenly the hammer paused in mid-air and Carmen spun round, as if she had sensed my presence.

'Who are you looking for?'

'Madame Avril?'

'Yes?'

My heart began pounding as I delivered, as naturally as possible, the speech that I had practised in my head ten times over since Yport.

'I'm Captain Lopez. Fécamp police station. I'd like to talk to you.'

She looked me up and down. A question seemed to be burning on her lips – 'They're recruiting cripples in the police these days?' – but she managed to restrain herself.

'What do you want from me?'

'I'll get right to the point, Madame Avril. It's about the murder of your daughter, Morgane. Something . . . something new has come up.'

The hammer crashed to the tiles of the terrace before Carmen could stop it. Her red face, as faded as an apple forgotten at the bottom of a basket, seemed to crack. Relief flooded through me.

Piroz hadn't contacted her!

Which was odd, given the number of similarities between Magali Verron and Morgane Avril, but I'd been gambling on Carmen Avril not having heard from the police.

'Something new?'

'Nothing concrete, Madame Avril, I don't want to raise any false hopes. But a series of disturbing events have taken place in Yport over the last few days. Can I come in?'

The interior of the building was level with the landscaped garden. With its exposed beams, a fireplace in which you could have roasted a calf, and rustic touches like the old cartwheel that had been converted into a table, it was the perfect rustic setting for tourists passing through the area.

Carmen invited me to take a seat on a sofa that smelled of leather. For a moment I wondered how a woman had managed to keep this place running single-handed. Then I launched into my account of everything that had happened.

The suicide of Magali Verron, the rape that preceded it, the Burberry cashmere scarf found around her neck.

I omitted to mention one detail: that Magali had bumped into a jogger at the top of the cliff.

Carmen Avril listened to me open-mouthed for almost a quarter of an hour.

'The bastard's back,' she muttered between her teeth.

I took from my rucksack the 'Magali Verron' file that I had stolen from Piroz's office. The red, white and blue headers and official stamps lent credibility to the information that I was about to give Carmen.

'You'll have to listen to me without interrupting, Madame Avril. Only then will I ask you for an explanation. If you have one . . .'

She nodded excitedly. Her daughter's killer had resurfaced, she was willing to listen to anything. I took a deep breath and listed all the things I had learned about Magali Verron.

Born on 10 May 1993, in Neufchâtel, Canada. Attended school in the Paris region, at the Claude Monet primary school, Albert Schweitzer middle school and Georges Brassens upper school, before going on to become a medical student. *Raqs sharqi* dancer. Fan of seventies rock.

Carmen's excitement turned into bafflement.

What could be the meaning of this? The same birthday as her

daughter, born in a town of the same name, attending schools of the same name, sharing the same tastes.

Sheer insanity.

Carmen Avril rose to her feet without a word; only a slight imbalance in her gait betrayed the effect my words had had on her. She went to the kitchenette and returned with a 'welcome' tray, the sort she might offer her guests. Local biscuits, glasses, a jug of water, orange juice and cold milk. The tray vibrated in her trembling hands. She set it down on the low table before addressing me in a hesitant voice.

'Captain Lopez, what can I say? Everything you have told me seems incredible. Absolutely incredible. Who is this girl? This . . . Magali Verron?'

I poured myself a glass of milk before delivering my next bombshell.

'I haven't yet told you everything, Madame Avril. Magali Verron looked like your daughter. A most unsettling resemblance—'

I was debating whether to bring up the in vitro fertilisation of her daughter, and the possibility that Morgane and Magali might have been half-sisters, via their father. Carmen, as if reading my thoughts, cut in:

'A resemblance, Captain Lopez? That's ridiculous. Morgane didn't have a younger sister! And neither did she have a cousin ten years younger than her. Just me and her sister Océane.'

I shook my head as if trying to come up with another possible explanation. In truth, I was playing for time. If I was going to catch this fish, I would need to reel her in slowly. I flicked through the 'Magali Verron' file again, to the page with details of her DNA.

'Madame Avril, we know that you are the keeper of the Fil Rouge Association's archives. I've come here today because there's something I need to check with you.'

Carmen was bound to take the bait. If all I had read about her was true, she would be ready to pursue any trail that might lead her to her daughter's murderer. However far-fetched it might sound.

I carelessly picked up a biscuit, and then pushed the page towards her.

'I'd like to compare Magali Verron's DNA with Morgane's.'

The line went taut. Carmen's voice hardened. For ten years, she had learned to be suspicious of the police.

'You didn't keep my daughter's file in your own archives?'

I flailed for a second.

'Yes. Yes, of course. But to access that file would involve a lengthy bureaucratic procedure, obtaining the permission of the examining magistrate and various other parties. I thought it would be quicker to come straight to you.'

I couldn't tell from her expression whether she believed me. I was hoping she would seize upon my explanation as further proof of the incompetence of the police.

'Do you work with Captain Piroz?' she asked.

I went on steadily chewing the biscuit. Honey and almond. Slightly sticky. On the way to Neufchâtel I had run through all the possible question in my head, but stupidly I hadn't predicted that one.

I swallowed, buying a few more seconds to decide on my answer.

'Yes, of course. He sent me here.'

Her cheeks flushed crimson. For the first time Carmen Avril seemed to be relax.

'OK, come with me to the office. Piroz is the only honest police-man in Normandy.'

I wasn't about to tell her I didn't share her opinion. She led me into an office, then commanded,

'Wait for me here.'

Madame Avril disappeared into an adjoining room, presumably the one where she archived all her information about the Avril–Camus case. During her absence I took a good around me. It seemed to be a nursery that Carmen had converted into an office. The wallpaper pattern was made up of aeroplanes and balloons. Everywhere I looked there were pictures of Morgane as a child. Morgane playing at being a doctor. Morgane playing at being a cowboy. Morgane playing at being a fireman.

Strangely, I didn't see a single photograph of her sister Océane.

Carmen returned with a box that she set down on a table balanced on a pair of trestles.

'I will leave that here for you to consult, Captain, and I'll be back with you in a minute.'

She disappeared into the adjacent room again while I pounced on the box. After feverishly flicking through some loose pages, I stopped on the photocopy of a document from Fécamp police station.

DNA results – Morgane Avril – Monday, 7 June 2004 – Regional Forensic Service, Rouen

I set the other page down alongside it. The presentation and the font used by the regional crime squad had changed since 2014, but the logos, the headed paper and the stamps were the same.

DNA results – Magali Verron – Thursday, 20 February 2014 – Regional Forensic Service, Rouen

The first column indicated blood group. Both Morgane and Magali were group B+. Not the most common group, from what I remembered of the biology course I had taken at the Saint Antoine Institute. Less than ten per cent of the French population.

Another coincidence.

Shivers ran down the back of my neck. My eyes fell to the figures that made up the genetic code of the two girls.

I stopped on two graphics, annotated with long series of letters and numbers.

TH01 chr 11 6/9. D2 25/29. D 18 16/18
TH01 chr 11 6/9. D2 25/29. D 18 16/18

I ignored the details. Something to do with monozygotic and heterozygotic genotypes that I'd never understood, but I remembered that it was scientifically impossible for two different individuals to have the same markers and frequencies of occurrence. The figures danced in front of my eyes.

VWA chr 12 14/17 TPOX chr 15 9/12 FGA 21/23
VWA chr 12 14/17 TPOX chr 15 9/12 FGA 21/23

The green and blue curves looked like encephalograms, with an accuracy of a tenth of a millimetre. I could have gone on trying to find the slightest difference between the two histograms, but I had already understood . . .

Magali and Morgane's genetic profiles were identical!

I went on mechanically following the lines with the tip of my index finger, like a mad scientist endlessly rereading a formula that defied the laws of the universe.

D7 9/10. D16, 11/13, CSF1PO chr, 14/17
D7 9/10. D16, 11/13, CSF1PO chr, 14/17

What I was looking at was impossible.

Two individuals, born ten years apart, could not have the same genetic code!

Magali.

Morgane.

Were the two women one and the same?

As insane as the evidence appeared, that had been my conviction since the outset. Morgane Avril hadn't died ten years ago. She was the one who had spoken to me on Wednesday morning, near the blockhouse, before throwing herself off the cliff. Moreoever, as I considered the startling resemblance between Morgane Avril and the girl who had killed herself in front of my eyes, Magali Verron, it occurred to me that she had seemed a little older than the Morgane in the photographs from 2004. The same face, feature for feature, but a few years older, perhaps as many as ten.

Which brought me back to the same conclusion, even more obvious now: Morgane Avril was alive until two days ago!

Allele frequency D3, 0.0789. Genotype frequency D3, 0.013
Allele frequency D3, 0.0789. Genotype frequency D3, 0.013

I thought again of the huge legal machinery that had been put in place to solve the Avril case. The police, the judges, the witnesses, the journalists, the hundreds of newspaper articles. How had Morgane been able to deceive everyone? To survive? None of it made sense . . .

I went into the adjoining room to tell Carmen.

Her daughter Morgane, alive.

Only two days ago.

Before dying a second . . .

The proprietor of Dos-d'Âne hadn't heard me come in. She had her back towards me and was talking on the phone, covering her mouth and the receiver with her left hand.

'I'm telling you, I've got a colleague of yours here,' she whispered. 'For God's sake, Piroz, what is this nonsense about a lookalike of my daughter committing suicide in Yport the day before yesterday?'

My muscles tensed.

Carmen Avril was talking to the police!

The old bag had wanted to check up on me. She'd told me there was only one cop she trusted: Piroz.

Fuck!

I cursed myself for not being more vigilant. I took a step forward and pressed the speaker button on the base of the cordless phone.

Captain Piroz's hysterical voice exploded in the room.

'Keep him there, Madame Avril. Keep him there, damn it, we're on our way!'

Click.

My thumb ended the call. At that moment, almost without thinking, I took from my pocket the King Cobra I had borrowed from Mona's thesis supervisor and aimed it at Carmen.

'Who are you?' she yelled.

What was I supposed to do now?

Hold those DNA results in front of her until she believed me?

215

Leave her there and run, outside. And then run some more.

Where to?

Was there any escape from this spider's web? Wouldn't it be easier to set the revolver down and wait for Piroz on the living-room sofa?

Carmen leaned forward slightly, muscles taut, like a she-bear ready to leap out of her cave. The walls trembled around me, I struggled to keep the barrel of the King Cobra steady. The room we were standing in was a second nursery, which had been turned into a box room. Photographs of Morgane hung on the walls.

Morgane, three years old, draping Christmas garlands over her mother's shoulders.

Morgane, six years old, on a tractor.

Morgane, seven years old, climbing in the apple tree in the garden.

Carmen moved forward slightly. The barrel of the King Cobra lowered by a few millimetres, while my eye, on the photograph, moved down to another branch of the apple tree.

It was as if all my thoughts and suspicions had suddenly accelerated, bringing them into a headlong collision with my certainties. Then everything exploded in a thousand fragments of shrapnel.

I understood. Everything.

I knew who Magali Verron was . . .

Still clutching the butt of the King Cobra, I couldn't help letting out a long laugh, the laugh of a madman.

27

Who are you?

Two seven-year-old girls were balancing in the branches of the apple tree.

Morgane and her sister, Océane.

The same red caps, the same green coats with fur hoods, the same lined boots, the same woollen scarves around their necks.

The same age. The same face.

Twins!

As I wiped the corners of my eyes, wet with the tears of my nervous laugh, I raised the barrel of the King Cobra towards Carmen, gesturing to her not to try anything.

Morgane had a twin sister!

There had been no mention of that detail in the brown envelopes. Océane, the victim's sister, had given a statement after the Riff on the Cliff festival, but her age was never mentioned. I hadn't given it a second thought.

Now it was all clear.

They had omitted that information so that they could trap me more easily.

With the end of the revolver I beckoned to Carmen to leave the room.

In my head, several pieces of the puzzle were fitting together. Morgane had died, having been raped and murdered, on 5 June 2004. Ten years later it was Océane, her twin sister, who had thrown herself from the top of Yport cliff. It was her desperate expression that I had seen near the blockhouse. Océane probably couldn't cope with the death of her sister. So she had devised and acted the character of Magali Verron. The same birthday, the same tastes, the same education . . . And the same DNA!

I pushed Carmen towards the office. With my left hand I picked up the two sets of DNA results.

How had Océane been able to deceive the police? How had she managed to make everyone think that her virtual double, Magali Verron, was born ten years later, in Canada, and that she had lived there until the age of seven?

My eyes glided to the official stamp of the national police service.

Unless Piroz had deliberately fed me false information.

With the end of the revolver, I pointed to one of the photographs on the wall. The one in which a six-year-old girl was dressed up as a cowboy.

'Is that her?' I asked Carmen. 'Is that Océane, your other daughter?'

'Yes. They were inseparable. Océane was a tomboy, Morgane a little princess, but no one could come between them, not even me. When Morgane was murdered, I didn't think Océane would survive her.'

'For ten years, at least,' I said. 'It was Océane, wasn't it – she was the one who threw herself off the cliff two days ago?'

As I said those words, I realised that something didn't add up. Carmen Avril was watching me suspiciously, but I saw no sadness or anger in her attitude. Nothing to suggest that she had just lost her second daughter in a tragedy very like the one that had occurred ten years ago.

She turned her head towards the clock hanging over the door.

'Do I look like a grieving mother?'

I thought of the words that Piroz had yelled down the telephone. *Keep him there, for God's sake, we're on our way.*

I had to get out of there as quickly as possible. But I heard myself answering calmly, separating the words to give them equal importance.

'It was your daughter, Madame Avril. It was Océane. I saw her jumping. I . . . I saw her corpse.'

The proprietor of the Dos-d'Âne smiled at me. Far from shocked. 'When was that?'

'Wednesday. Two days ago. Early in the morning . . .'

'I find that hard to believe, monsieur . . . Lopez.'

She stepped forward, and my revolver came level with her belly. 'I spoke to Océane on the phone, less than five hours ago.'

She had to be bluffing.

Carmen Avril was lying. To give Piroz time to get there. They all wanted to pin the deaths of the three girls on me.

'OK, I believe you,' I said at last. 'Your daughter Océane is alive, she didn't throw herself off the cliff at Yport the day before yesterday. But in that case, I want to talk to her.'

'Out of the question!'

'Does she live far from here?'

Carmen gave me a contemptuous look. 'You're a dangerous mental patient who needs to be locked up.'

I was running out of time. Piroz, or the police from Neufchâtel, would be here any minute.

'You have no idea how dangerous, Madame Avril. Right now I need to get out of here, and you're coming with me.'

Seeing my determination, she obeyed without protest. She walked into the garden, the gravel crunching under her feet. The apple tree cast its shadow over the frosty grass. At every moment, I imagined I could hear the police siren ripping through the silence, or squad cars speeding down the drive.

But the Foucarmont road was deserted. Carmen Avril got into the passenger seat of the Fiat 500. I was still holding the revolver, but even so I found her astonishingly cooperative.

'Don't try to get away,' I warned her, as I put the key in the ignition.

'You needn't worry about that. I don't know who you are, but you're somehow connected to Morgane's death. And the death of the girl who was raped and strangled the day before yesterday.'

'Raped perhaps. But not strangled.'

She looked at me as if I were a child she had caught in a lie.

'Strangled! Piroz told me a moment ago. This girl Magali Verron didn't kill herself as you told me, she was murdered. I'm not about to let you go, Lopez – I've been waiting ten years for this moment . . .'

What moment?

Before I could put the question, Carmen delivered the answer.

'For the murderer of my daughter and little Myrtille Camus to strike again.'

I held her gaze.

'Piroz is playing a dirty game. I don't know what he's told you, but he's looking for a scapegoat. Well, he's out of luck, because he's not going to pin any of this on me.'

Carmen shrugged as if my words carried no weight. It didn't matter, she was prepared to come with me. Her quest for the truth was more important to her than her own safety.

'Where are you taking me?'

I started the car without replying. We drove two kilometres to get out of Neufchâtel, then I turned on to a dirt road. 'Green avenue, access no. 11', according to the wooden sign. I parked under a lime tree after the first turning. I switched off the engine and aimed the King Cobra at my passenger again.

'Give me your phone. Now.'

'What for?'

Carmen didn't move either to help me or to protest when I leaned over to grab her handbag and take out a Samsung Galaxy.

My thumb slid over the touch screen.

List of contacts.

OCÉANE.

I double-clicked to call her.

Océane's photograph appeared. Full screen. An electric shock!

It was her, no question about it.

Magali Verron and Océane Avril were one and the same.

In the picture on the phone she was smiling under a cotton-wool sky, in a pose almost identical to the one she had adopted a second before jumping off the cliff, her tousled hair blowing in the wind, her eyes narrowed to an almond shape, staring into the sun as if defying the light.

Just before she crashed on to the pebbles. The girl whose telephone number I was dialling had died, two days ago.

A voice answered at the first ring. A distant whisper, almost inaudible.

'Mum? I'm in the middle of a consultation. I'll call you back in ten minutes.'

I waited in silence for a few moments before working out that she had already hung up.

On the passenger seat, Carmen was looking triumphant.

'Happy now, Lopez? You've heard Océane's voice. You didn't find yourself talking to a ghost's answering machine? You didn't dial the number of heaven?'

The Samsung slipped between my sweating hands. I had stopped thinking. My brain was ready to implode. Then it hit me: I had no proof that the girl who'd answered the phone was Océane Avril! The list of contacts ran past under my fingers. I stopped a few letters further down.

OCÉANE WORK

Double click.

Three rings this time before anyone picked up: a cheerful woman's voice, talking loudly and articulating each word.

'Marquis Medical Centre, hello.'

I breathed for a few seconds, then improvised.

'Hello! I've been trying to get hold of you for ages. I have an appointment at the hospital in a quarter of an hour. Can you tell me how to get there?'

'No problem, monsieur, are you in Neufchâtel?'

'Almost . . .'

Carmen rolled panicked eyes as the secretary told me the way.

Turn towards the centre of town, right towards the main street, right again before you get to the church. After waking up briefly while the children got out of school, Neufchâtel seemed to have fallen back into a cold and dusty damp.

No trace of the police.

The Place du Marquis was almost empty. I parked right outside the surgery.

In spite of the revolver pointed at her, Carmen was reluctant to get out of the Fiat. For the first time I read something like fear on her face. I gripped the King Cobra, stammering some words that sounded like an apology.

'I haven't killed anyone, Carmen. I just want to know the truth. Like you.'

She spat her reply: 'She won't be the one you're expecting, Lopez. Océane works on the other side of this door. She isn't the girl you're looking for, this Magali Verron that you couldn't save.'

Resigned, she unfastened her seat belt, then added: 'Not her, and no other daughter of mine. I assure you, I didn't have triplets . . .'

I had thought of that possibility for a moment.

Triplets, quadruplets, quintuplets.

Identical clones, jumping off the cliff one after another. One every ten years. Ridiculous! A plot from a cheap thriller.

I checked that the car park was deserted, then got out of the Fiat, being careful to hide my wrist and the revolver under a dirty rag that I had dug out of the glove compartment. To a passer-by in a hurry it might have looked like a makeshift bandage.

I pushed the polished glass door and let Carmen walk in ahead of me. I took in the four gilded plaques engraved with the names and titles of the doctors who worked at the surgery. I stopped at the third.

Océane Avril
Gynaecologist obstetrician.

My prosthesis slipped on the step. I regained my balance by leaning against the wall, without letting go of the gun hidden under the rag in my hand.

No! a voice yelled in my head. The girl who had just taken my call on the phone couldn't have been Morgane's twin sister. Her twin sister had fallen 120 metres, right in front of my eyes. As if clinging to a pair of crutches, I relied on the two axioms Mona had put forward the previous evening. The only two certainties.

Morgane Avril died ten years ago.

Magali Verron died two days ago.

Their incredible resemblance, even their identical genetic imprints, could only be explained by the fact that they were twins.

I entered the clinic and, with a gesture that might have looked friendly, rested my bandaged hand against Carmen's hip. A girl in a white coat smiled at us from behind the reception desk, then addressed Carmen directly.

'Hello, Madame Avril. If you want to see Océane, she's in a meeting. She shouldn't be long.'

She stared at the door to my right.

Doctor Avril.

Without thinking, I let go of Carmen and pushed the door.

Four pairs of eyes were aimed at me.

A woman sitting down, holding her round belly between her trembling palms.

A man standing beside her, with his hand on her shoulder, the other one ready to hit anyone who came too close.

In the corner of the room a two-year-old child was playing on all fours with a shaky Lego tower.

And Océane Avril, behind her desk.

'Can I help you?'

The obstetrician studied me without understanding my intrusion.

A wave of heat overwhelmed me.

It was her . . . It was Magali Verron.

The same melancholy expression. The same delicate grace.

The same perfect features, as if a painter had drawn her to my specifications – the girl of my dreams. How could I have been mistaken?

The one I had reached out to on the cliffs by the blockhouse.

The one whose corpse I had stood over on the beach, for many long minutes before the Fécamp police arrived.

The one standing in front of me. Plainly alive, and explaining to a young couple how to bring a child into the world . . .

My arm dangled stupidly. The rag fell to the ground like a dead jellyfish, revealing the King Cobra.

The pregnant woman screamed, making her son cry. The Lego tower toppled. The child ran across the room and jumped up to press himself against his father's torso. Jaw firm. Fists clenched.

'Get out of here!' Océane ordered.

Carmen Avril was standing between the door and the corridor, blocking my exit. Naked babies of all skin colours stared at me from their glass frames on all the walls, indignant, closing in on me.

I had to flee. And then think.

I spun round and pushed Carmen with all my strength. She fell backwards, knocking over two chairs in the corridor. I waved the revolver in front of me, which prompted more screaming, this time from the girl in the white coat at reception.

The glass door flew open.

One second later, I was behind the wheel of the Fiat 500. Another second and the car reversed into the empty car park, turned and screeched into the main road, ignoring the stop sign.

I got my breath back and forced myself to take my foot off the accelerator, to drive slowly, at least until the Neufchâtel exit. In my rear-view mirror, down by the Foucarmont road, I thought I saw the blue halo of a revolving light, just below the panel that said 'Gîtes de France'.

I slowed down . . .

The cops were at Carmen's place!

It would probably be a while before they had my description, the make of my car, perhaps even the detail of the mineralogical sticker on the window, if Carmen had been observant.

The Fiat crossed the Arques bridge: '49 km/h,' said a luminous smiley face.

I needed to disappear. Carmen might already have called the police. If they missed me in Neufchâtel, they were bound to be waiting to catch me on the motorway.

I turned right towards Mesnières-en-Bray. Country roads would be my best option.

I had one chance.

The police weren't about to launch a national manhunt. I didn't know the procedures involved, but it wasn't something they seemed to do when it was just an everyday murderer on the run. If I stuck to secondary roads, if I waited for nightfall, with a bit of luck I'd be able to get back to Vaucottes.

And then . . .

I turned on the headlights. The road stretched out ahead of me. In the gloom, the white line in the middle of the road quickly became my only point of reference. A thread of Ariadne that divided my path into two equal parts. My eyes concentrated on that line, hypnotised, as if by continuing to stare at it I might split my reason into two watertight chambers.

The first one ran out. I had invented everything. No girl had committed suicide two days ago. If that girl existed, she had been strangled to death by my very hands. Her face wasn't the face of Océane Avril, I'd got muddled up with another murder, ten years earlier, the murder of her sister. Perhaps I had strangled Morgane as well. I was mad, I killed, I forgot, I couldn't tell my victims apart. I didn't remember Myrtille Camus either, but if I had murdered Morgane Avril, I must also have raped and murdered this third girl.

The white strip in the glaring light of the headlights rolled out slowly, dizzyingly.

Now I understood those innocent people who confess to crimes they haven't committed, after nights in custody, after hours of arguments, hypotheses and evidence hurled at them by the prosecution. Those innocent people who end up believing in the truth set out by other people, who end up doubting their own certainties, the ones they had when they came into the judge's office.

A sharp turn.

The alabaster line turned in a hairpin bend.

No! the voice roared in my head.

No!

The second chamber of my reason continued to resist. There must be a key, a logical explanation.

It was there, almost within reach.

All I had to do was calm down and think. Collect all the evidence and put it together in a different way.

I needed to get some distance, examine it from a new perspective. Go beyond appearances.

Talk to someone who would believe me.

Mona?

28

Talk to someone who would believe me?

'Do the police have a description of my car?'

Mona was yelling down the phone.

The headlights of the Fiat blinded a little boy who was about to run into the road, a ball under his arm, just before the sign that read 'Carville-Pot-de-Fer'.

I slammed on the brakes. The sign beside the boy taunted me: 'Slow down, think of our children'. The cardboard child watched me slowly pass by with great indifference.

Carville-Pot-de-Fer was asleep.

For almost an hour I had been jumping from one village to another along muddy side roads as uneven as the trenches of the Pays de Caux.

'I'm not sure, Mona. Carmen Avril may not have noticed the sticker.'

'You think so? When she's been waiting for her daughter's murderer for ten years? Christ, Jamal, the cops are going to make the connection with me as soon as she talks to them about a Fiat 500.'

The twin brother of the little boy with the ball was already getting smaller in my rear-view mirror. Carville-Pot-de-Fer had turned out to be nothing more than a hamlet. I should have told Mona to let it go, tell the police I had stolen her car, that the door didn't shut, that . . .

'Come and see me in Vaucottes,' I murmured into the phone.

'And how do I do that? You're driving my car.'

I was reluctant to suggest a meeting point near Yport. Too risky.

'On foot? It's barely two kilometres to Vaucottes.'

For a moment I thought Mona was going to hang up on me. A huge mansion house, lights blazing, came into view on the crest overlooking the Durdent Valley.

'Two kilometres! And what about that cliff I'll have to climb up and back down again? I haven't got a bionic leg, unlike some people!'

The rain started falling at about nine in the evening. Cold and dense. I imagined it must be turning into snow a few miles inland. In the Valleuse de Caucottes, it merely ran down the tarmacked slope, forming a fleeting torrent which would then spill over the pebbles. An *oued*, my mother would have called it. A wadi. Was there a local synonym?

I kept watch at the window for Mona. Several times I thought of going outside, of getting back into the car parked in Martin Denain's garden and going to find her. But Mona would probably take the coastal path . . . What was the point of taking an additional risk? To salve my guilty conscience?

Twenty minutes later, a beam of light pierced the rain, shyly and hesitantly. A dark silhouette advanced behind it, braced against the wind and the pelting rain. I still thought of hurrying outside, opening the door, holding out a blanket and calling into the night, 'My God, you came!'

But was it Mona coming into the garden?

I didn't recognise her until she threw open the oak door. At first Mona didn't say a word, she just pulled off the waterproof yellow cape that made her look like an elf and pressed it, soaking, against my chest.

I left it to drip on the parquet. I noticed that, for the first time since yesterday, Mona wasn't wearing my sheriff's star pinned to her heart. I assumed she was going to start by yelling at me. After that she would listen to me.

Mona stared at me for a long time. I thought how pretty she was, with her red hair sticking to her streaming face, like a little woodland creature escaping the storm to find refuge in the house in the clearing. Fearful. The kind you wanted to press to your heart to warm it up. Then she gave that irresistible smile.

'I don't think anyone followed me!'

She closed the door on the rainstorm.

'I'm going to take a shower, Jamal. A really hot shower.'

Mona came back down half an hour later. She had taken off all her wet clothes and pulled over her naked skin a big grey woollen pullover that came to halfway down her thigh and slipped down over her right shoulder. Her red hair was combed back, exposing her forehead. She sat down on the sofa, pulled the jumper down until it covered her bare thighs, which were drawn up against her chest, then gave me a questioning look.

'So, tell me.'

I told her the whole story.

My trip to Neufchâtel-en-Bray to find Carmen Avril. My ruse to make her dig out the police file on Morgane. The matching DNA. The photographs of the twin sisters. The race to the doctor's surgery. My face-to-face encounter with Océane Avril. Alive . . .

'Was she as beautiful as she was in your memory?'

I was taken aback by the question. I didn't reply. Not really.

'It was her, Mona. Even if I know it's impossible, it was her. The girl who went by the name of Magali Verron. The one I held out the scarf to on the cliff before she jumped.'

She didn't press the point. She asked me to make her some tea. I found some Twinings bags under Denain's sink. When I came back into the room, she was gripping both her legs between her arms, with her chin resting on her knees like a hedgehog curled up in a ball.

'You're still not thinking of handing yourself in to the cops?'

'They're trying to frame me, Mona.'

'OK, OK, let's not have that conversation again.'

'Thanks for coming.'

'My pleasure. Thanks for the adrenaline.'

The kettle whistled in the kitchen. I didn't move.

'What are you going to do now?' Mona asked.

'I was thinking on the way here. I'm giving myself one night. Just one night. We'll start over from the beginning, we'll look for a solution, a way of fitting all the pieces together. If I haven't found it by tomorrow, I'll call Piroz and give myself up.'

Mona looked at the pendulum moving like a metronome in the case of the Norman clock.

9.40 p.m.

'A night? Deal! If we take off three hours to sleep for a bit, and at least one to make love, that doesn't leave us a lot of time . . .'

She got up. The XXL virgin wool sweater fell to the beginning of her white breasts. She put her bare feet on the brown parquet.

'Where shall we start?'

I replied without a moment's hesitation:

'Magali Verron! The police have been working for ten years on the Avril–Camus case, without finding much. This Magali Verron is the key to everything.'

I spread the two files out on the table, the one for Morgane Avril that I'd borrowed from her mother and the one for Magali Verron which I'd taken from Piroz's office.

'OK,' Mona said. 'I'll go on the internet. Perhaps you missed some information about her yesterday.'

She came over and pressed herself against me. She smelled of apple shower gel. My hands glided over her bare thighs, her warm bottom, her firm, curved waist beneath the thick wool. She stood on tiptoe as I pressed my erect penis against her belly. The woollen jumper was only a silk cocoon wrapping her body, which was there for the taking. At that moment it seemed big enough for us both to fit into it. Mona kissed me on the lips for a long time, then pushed me gently away.

'Time to work, big fella!'

She sat down at Martin Denain's computer. I took out some of the pages from the envelopes and spread them out across the table.

Concentrate.

We were like a couple of students frantically revising the night before an important exam.

230

The brass pendulum tapped out the passing of time, as if beating against the boards to escape its oak coffin.

Mona's exclamation ripped through the silence.

'Are you serious?'

I walked over, surprised. Leaning over her, my eye flicked from the laptop screen to her breasts, naked under her jumper.

'Yesterday,' Mona said with her head lowered, 'at the playground in Yport, you reconstructed Magali Verron's life on the basis of internet links. Facebook. Copains d'avant. Twitter. LinkedIn. Dailymotion. You remember? Two columns, one for Morgane, one for Magali. Pink Floyd et cetera – her favourite bands; her passion for *raqs sharqi*; her school in Canada, then middle school and upper school near Paris, with the same names as establishments in Neufchâtel-en-Bray. Everything, including her date of birth – the same day, the same place, ten years apart . . . That insane series of similarities.'

'Yes, and what have you found?'

Mona looked at me sadly. Like when you have to tell a six-year-old about the death of one of its parents.

'Nothing, Jamal. There's nothing on the internet. I've tried all the search engines, there's no trace of Magali Verron. It's as if she never existed.'

29

As if she never existed?

My fingers sped across the keyboard like those of a crazed pianist. I remembered the routes I had followed to dig out information about Magali Verron. Sites accessible in three clicks, on which millions of young adults set out their lives.

Nothing.

There was no longer any trace of the girl on the web.

I turned to Mona.

'Someone's deleted all the information . . .'

My voice trembled. Mona didn't say anything, so I added:

'Anyone can do that. Delete internet pages. It's just more proof . . .' I held my breath. 'More proof that they're trying to trap me.'

Mona stood up. She pulled her jumper down to halfway along her thigh, but the wool climbed back up again, revealing gooseflesh on her skin.

'What if you imagined the girl?'

I looked at Mona without a word. She was walking back and forth in the room, barefoot, unable to stay still for a second.

'My God, Jamal! What do we know about Magali Verron? Only what you've told me! You say you've read about her life on the net, but there's nothing there about her. You described her face to me, but it's the face of another girl, a girl who died ten years ago, or her living twin. You say that girl threw herself from the cliff, raped, strangled, but the media hasn't reported it. No other eye-witness can confirm it. Your Christian Le Medef has disappeared.

232

Denise Joubain claims she hasn't left her house in months . . . Do you see, Jamal! You've made it all up. There was no suicide three days ago. You imagined the scene! You imagined the face of that girl. You imagined her life. You imagined those witnesses.'

I leapt to my feet. I waved under Mona's nose the file I had stolen from Piroz's office.

A green folder.

Magali Verron, written in black felt tip, in Piroz's handwriting.

'And what about the police who are after me? Did I imagine their accusations too? The cops came to see you this morning at the Sirène, isn't that right?'

She replied with the patience of a schoolteacher.

'Exactly. The police were looking for you. They stayed for two minutes, they asked me if I knew you, if I knew where you were, but they never once mentioned Magali Verron. Nothing about a rape the day before yesterday.'

I held the file up in front of her eyes.

'Shit, Mona! What about the medical reports? And the photographs of Magali Verron's disjointed limbs, and those DNA results with the police stamp on them? Am I so crazy that I made those up?'

For the first time she seemed to be filled with doubt.

'I don't know. All I can see is that, if you made it all up, that explains everything. Almost everything . . . And then, more importantly, it would be good news, wouldn't it?'

Good news?

I stared at her, perplexed.

'Think about it, Jamal. If there was no corpse, no Magali Verron, that means there was no rape. No accusation of murder. The police have nothing on you! You're just a bit paranoid, perhaps you embellished things a little to get me into bed . . .'

'Damn it, Mona, what would I have been doing at the police station the day we met by the drinks machine?'

'I have no idea. Perhaps they'd brought you in as a witness for something else . . .'

She paused.

Suddenly I understood.

I saw the other side of the piece of the puzzle put in place by Mona.

I hadn't imagined Magali Verron. Her face, her rape, the red scarf around her neck, the cliffs of Yport.

I was seeing again a scene that I had witnessed before!

That was probably what Mona thought. The police in Fécamp had called me in as a witness to a ten-year-old case: the murder of Morgane Avril. I had somehow mixed up the past with an imagined present.

I was insane . . .

Still clinging to the precipice, desperate to save myself from falling over the edge, I pointed to the documents on the table.

'What about the envelopes?' I asked Mona, 'Did I send them to myself?'

She came over and rested her hand on my shoulder.

'No, Jamal. No. But might it be someone who's trying to make you remember about the Avril–Camus case? That would explain . . .'

I pushed her hand away.

'Make me remember what? I'd never heard of that case before this week!'

Mona put her hand under her jumper. I immediately regretted my reaction. I no longer knew where I was. Guilty or innocent? My eyes stung and I wanted to cry. To burst into tears like a child.

'I . . . I have nothing to do with this case, Mona. They're trying to pin it on me. They're trying to drive me mad. If you leave me on my own, they'll do it.'

Mona took her eyes off mine and stared at the clock one last time: 10.10 p.m.

'One night, Jamal! I'm giving you one night to convince me. As soon as the sun appears over the cliffs, you're going to the station.'

'And between now and then, do I get to decide the battle plan?'

'Go on.'

'Apart from Piroz and the police, only two people can confirm that I didn't make up the suicide of Magali Verron: Christian Le Medef and Denise Joubain.'

'You've already questioned them.'

Yes, Le Medef confirmed everything before he disappeared. Or before they made him disappear. Denise Joubain was terrified. If we go back to both their houses you can make your own mind up.'

'In the middle of the night?'

'Yes.'

'What about the police? You might bump into them in Yport.'

'Cops on my heels? Don't you think you're being a bit paranoid?'

Mona burst out laughing. Her lips brushed against mine.

'Weren't you going to make me some tea?'

I saw her going towards the kitchen. I exclaimed:

'In my defence, will you allow me to call a friend?'

'I'm sorry?'

'There is another trail that I haven't followed, that sequence of numbers that I found in Piroz's office and at Le Medef's. Impossible to find anything on the internet that has anything to do with them. I have a friend with a brain like an encyclopaedia at the Saint Antoine Institute. Ibou. You never know . . .'

'You're right, call a clever friend, what do research chemists know about anything?'

Ibou replied almost immediately. I cut short his questions about my training for the North Face, about the local weather and the latest gossip from the Institute.

'Can you spare me a minute, Ibou? You have nothing to gain, but you might help me out of a hole . . .'

I set the scene, I listed the figures, convinced that it was an impossible code to break.

2/2	3/0
0/3	1/1

Ibou's loud laughter echoed down the line.

'Easy peasy, my little bunny rabbit. Everyone knows that one! It's the square of the prisoner's dilemma.'

'The what?'

'The prisoner's dilemma! It's game theory.'

I turned on the speaker so that Mona could hear.

'The principle is simple. Imagine that two suspects, of a robbery, for example, are arrested by the police and interrogated separately. Each prisoner, if he doesn't want to confess to the crime, has two options: to say nothing or to accuse his accomplice. If he accuses him, he will get a reduction in his sentence and his friend will get the maximum. But the problem is that neither prisoner knows what the other one is going to do . . .'

'I don't understand, Ibou. Where do those numbers fit into this story of yours?'

'I'm getting to that. The numbers represent the outcome: years in prison, for example. If the two prisoners say nothing, they'll be given the benefit of the doubt and get one year in prison each. If they accuse each other, they both go down and get two years in prison.'

'So why talk to the cops in the first place?'

'Because if the theorem is to work at all, individual interest must outweigh cooperative interest. If one of the prisoners accuses the other without himself being betrayed, he is cleared and the other receives the full weight of the law, three years in jail for his friend and zero for himself. He's free!'

'Holy shit, Ibou. Do they really pay researchers to come up with this stuff?'

'Yes! An American called Robert Axelrod ran a competition to find the equation that would allow players to win maximum points in the game of the prisoner's dilemma.'

'You can play it?'

'Yes. Two players. Ten. A hundred. The rule is the simplest in the world: you betray, or you cooperate. You make your choice in secret and then you compare it with what the other players have done and you count up the points.'

'And after that? What's the magic formula?'

According to Axelrod, it's summed up in three words. Cooper-ation–reciprocity–pardon. In short, first you suggest cooperation to

236

another player. If he fucks you over and betrays you, next thing you do is betray him right back. Then you propose cooperation again. According to Axelrod, it's the golden rule that should influence all behavioural interactions between human beings.'

'And that's it?'

I couldn't see a connection between this idiotic theory, the Avril–Camus case and the suicide of Magali Verron. Why had Piroz and Le Medef written the numbers of that theorem down on a piece of paper?

I thought for a few seconds.

'Tell me if I'm wrong, Ibou, but this guy Axelrod's solution only works if the players play against one another several times. The principle is not to allow yourself to be fucked over twice in a row. But if you only play once, once and for all, the right answer is to win the confidence of the guy you're playing with and then betray him, is that it?'

'You've got it!'

I hung up without feeling that I'd made any progress. Clearly, the prisoner's dilemma didn't inspire Mona much either. Perhaps I'd made up those sequences of scribbled figures too . . .

Mona stuffed a packet of biscuits in a plastic bag, took out a thermos and turned on the coffee machine.

'You can't have slept for more than two hours since yesterday. Keep an eye on the coffee, I'm going to change.'

I immediately wondered where she was going to find dry women's clothes in this house, but she didn't give me time to think. She tugged nervously on her sweater.

'I need to know, Jamal. It's important . . .' She was still holding the wool, twisting its stitches out of shape. 'Ten years ago, did you . . .' The grey pullover was now nothing but a grille casting zebra shapes on her naked skin. 'Did you still have the use of both legs?'

The same question that Piroz asked me at the station.

I looked her up and down. Cynically. Icily.

'The use of both legs? Is that the question, Mona? Go on, then, pursue this thought to its conclusion. Was I able to dance ten years

237

ago? To climb cliffs? Run after a girl? Chat her up, rape her, strangle her, is that the question you're asking, Mona?'

'It's not what I think, Jamal.'

'They'd have spotted a cripple around the place.'

'I need you to tell me,' Mona said again.

I gently lifted my trouser leg to reveal the metal stem that connected my knee to my carbon foot.

'I crashed through the shop window at the Beaugrenelle shopping centre, in the fifteenth arrondissement. I was doing parkour with a group of about ten friends from La Courneuve. My fibular nerve was completely severed.'

Mona opened her mouth like a fish out of water. I was ahead of her.

'It happened in May 2002, twelve years ago.'

Mona didn't turn a hair. She let go of the jumper, which returned to its normal mohair shape.

'Are you pulling my leg?'

'Maybe, I love making up stories.'

Mona opted to drive. She had put on a pair of jeans, very fashionable but too big for her, probably borrowed from the wardrobe of Martin Denain's son, and a green pullover under her jacket, still damp from the rain.

Still no star pinned to her heart . . .

The rain had eased off, but the thermometer had fallen below zero. Before Mona started the car, I rested my fingers on her hand.

'If things go wrong . . .'

I opened the glove compartment. My hand touched the cold trigger of the King Cobra. I thought Mona was going to scream.

Quite the opposite!

She stared at me as if I was a complete idiot.

'Is that Martin Denain's revolver? It's a defensive weapon, Jamal! It only fires rubber bullets or blanks. Martin would never have kept a deadly weapon at his house.'

Was I reassured or terrified by Mona's revelation?

I didn't have time to think, since a moment later my fingers brushed against the sulphurised surface of some paper as I was putting the gun back. The texture of an envelope.

A brown envelope.

With my name on it.

It hadn't been in the glove compartment two hours before, when I had parked the Fiat at the end of the drive and put the King Cobra in there. Was it possible that some stranger, without making any noise, should have entered the garden, taking advantage of the darkness and the rain?

A stranger . . . or Mona?

Having decided to ask her for an explanation, I looked over at her . . . and understood that she was thinking the same thing.

For her, I was the only person who could have slipped the envelope into the car.

The only person who knew that I was going to open the glove compartment to take out the revolver.

Mona was still staring at me. I thought again of Ibou's words. The prisoner's dilemma.

That damned game . . .

Two accomplices. One secret choice.

Betray or trust.

Then I tore open the envelope.

30

Cooperation–reciprocity–pardon?

Diary of Alina Masson – December 2004

For as long as I can remember, Myrtille has always been there.

I lived on Rue Puchot, a sixth-floor apartment with a view of the Seine, the Pont Guynemer and the towpath where we never went to play.

Myrtille lived on the Passage Tabouelle, in a little town house with a small garden. Right on the street.

I always called her Mimy.

I was Lina.

Mimy–Lina.

The inseparable duo.

We worked out that we had first encountered one another at the Feugrains Hospital in 1983. I had left the maternity ward on December seventeenth, and Mimy was born there on the fifteenth. But her mother, Louise, liked to tell us that we had really become friends at the age of thirteen months, at the playground in Puchot, coming down the slide together in single file. I have often looked at the old photographs of the two of us, with our muffs, scarves and hats, since Mimy is no longer with us.

We met up again in the same class at nursery school. I often went to play at Mimy's house, with her and her mischievous little dog Buffo. I only found out much later that Charles had named it after a famous clown. We tormented the poor creature, we put him in the pram, we put bibs on him and gave him little pots of baby food to eat.

Mimy never came to mine. I was a little ashamed. And I didn't have a dog.

We were like a pair of twins, that was what they said about us at Alphonse Daudet primary school. Even if we didn't look like one another.

Louise and Charles worked very hard. Particularly on Wednesday, Saturday and during the holidays. Louise had her dance school, Charles did group tours of the museum. Sometimes we hung out in the street in Elbeuf, and most often we went to see Mimy's grandmother, Jeanine.

She lived on Route des Roches in Orival, in a house dug into the cliff of the Seine with grottoes in the garden that we weren't allowed to go to because of rockfalls. Jeanine made us laugh and wasn't very strict with us. We gave her the nickname Grandma Ninja.

Sometimes we took Buffo to her house. We kept him on a lead along the Boulevard de la Plage. The boulevard has always been called that, I think. But there hasn't been a beach on the banks of the Seine for as long as anyone can remember.

At the age of eight we went to our first summer camp together, in Bois-Plage-en-Ré, in the pines. Frédéric was already an activity leader, and Mimy thought he was incredibly handsome with his long hair, his guitar and muscular arms.

Louise and Charles ran the centre. The other kids gave Mimy hell because of it. She was the little princess, the bosses' daughter, maybe the only one whose parents both had jobs.

Mimy and I stood shoulder to shoulder.

Mimy–Lina, for ever.

At the Bois camp, as we called it, Mimy cried a lot and didn't want to tell her parents. We all slept together in a big dormitory. At night, Mimy sometimes wet the bed. She said as a joke that that was why the camp was called the Cloth of Gold, because of her pee-drenched sheets. I helped her. We arranged to be alone in the dormitory together and swapped mattresses. I lent her mine, and when one of our mattresses smelled too strongly of urine, we swapped it with the one belonging to the activity leader keeping watch in the corridor.

No one ever knew anything.

Our secret.

She would have killed me if I'd told anybody. I never said a word. She's the one who died.

After middle school, we met up again at the workshops in the community centre. Fred was there too. Mimy did dance and theatre. I just did circus skills. I was quite good at the tightrope, the balance ball, the barrel, the balance board, but Mimy was something else – perfect grace and harmony. Every now and then Louise would open the circus-theatre just for us and we'd walk about the round stage, dreaming. Once we found an old poster in the dressing room, a trapeze artist in a leotard, passing through a flaming hoop. His name was Rustam Trifon, and he was from a Moldavian circus. He was a beautiful as a god, fair-haired with eyes of steel. We put it up on our walls on alternate weeks. It drove us wild to have Rustam Trifon as an idol. He wasn't a bit like Filip Nikolic in 2B. We sang 'What's Up' by 4 Non Blondes as we dreamed of travelling the byways of Transnistria . . . That was where Rustam lived.

Our first camp as activity leaders in Bois-Plage-en-Ré was in 2001. Frédéric was the director, and Mimi still found him as handsome as ever, even with his hair cut very short and playing a ukulele. It was still the same kids from Elbeuf, or their cousins, their little brothers, perhaps even their children. Mimy and I thought it was hilarious when we got them up at night to go to the toilet, checking that their mattresses or pyjamas were dry.

We spent our wages on a trip to the Vieilles Charrues Festival the following year, and we saw the Blues Brothers. So close we could almost have touched them. We chatted up the Breton volunteers. They were gorgeous! One evening, Mimy went out with the one she said was the nicest of the lot, the one who cleaned the toilets.

Mimy was like that.

When we came back, after a fortnight in Finistère, Buffo was dead. On St Anne's day. He had just fallen asleep among the rose bushes, one afternoon when it was very hot. Charles buried him there: he dug a hole underneath him without even moving his body. Since then, every time I've called in on Charles and Louise at Impasse Tabouelle, I've never been able to look at the flowers without thinking of Buffo.

I think he'd have liked to be reincarnated as a rose.

In 2003, the camp left the Île de Ré for Normandy, because of funding cuts. We were also recruiting more teenagers. One evening in September, Mimy found a little lost puppy behind McDonald's in Caudebec-lès-Elbeuf. She called him Ronald, which was a bit of a stupid name, but it was the first clown's name she could think of. She carried him in her arms to Charles and Louise. That was a way of telling her parents that she wouldn't be there so much from now on. She had gone out with Fredéric during the camp. It was sort of inevitable, even if he was nineteen years older than she was.

We all expected it, to tell you the truth. We even thought they'd been pretty lucky to find one another. The next spring Mimy asked me if I wanted to be maid of honour at her wedding. She wanted it all to happen very quickly. The wedding was scheduled for 2 October in Orival, in the church on the banks of the Seine that was dug out of the cliff, as solid as her love, she said. Mimy was more romantic than me, and more Catholic too, more white dress, more poems, more Prince Charming.

I said yes. I also said I'd give her a hard time beforehand. That I was going to imagine the most mega-crazy events to celebrate the funeral of her time as a girl. In fact, I had planned for us both to go travelling after the camp in Isigny, for a month, to the other end of Europe, backpacking and hitch-hiking, perhaps all the way to Transnistria . . .

Mimy left me on 26 August 2004.

Without even saying goodbye.

It was her day off, and she'd never been further than the Chemin des Grandes Carrières, eight hundred metres from the camp in Isigny.

I was one of the first, with a police officer on either side of me, to discover her blue neck, her naked body under its torn dress, her wide eyes staring at the sky.

I was the one who told Charles and Louise. And they told Frédéric.

I ran through every minute of my life before calling them, at breakneck speed: the playground in Puchot, Buffo, the circus, Rustam Trifon, Grandma Ninja's grottoes . . .

I couldn't imagine spending the rest of my life without Mimy.

Charles, Louise, Frédéric and I wanted to know the truth.

But we didn't fit in with Carmen Avril and her Fil Rouge 'Never Forget' Association. Still, it was an opportunity to spend time talking to Océane, Morgane's sister. We were almost the same age, and we'd both lost the person dearest to us in the whole world.

Murdered by the same individual.

Twins of sorrow.

And yet we didn't understand each other. Not really. Like her mother, Océane was fuelled by hatred. Océane dreamed of finding her sister's murderer to kill her with her own bare hands. I think I might have been capable of going and visiting him every day in prison to tell him every detail of Mimy's life, to show him who she was, to make him regret his actions, so that he would love her and beg for her forgiveness.

Charles and Louise realised that we would never discover the truth about the death of their only daughter after the number one suspect, Olivier Roy, was identified.

And then cleared.

Commander Léo Bastinet informed them of the fact. Case closed . . . Barring any unexpected events. They left the Fil Rouge in 2005. It was their choice. They insisted that Frédéric and I should go on putting our energy into it.

Never forget.

At the time we didn't understand why.

Louise waited until December 2007, until the inauguration of the Elbeuf circus-theatre after ten years of renovation. Charles and Louise invited a number of major international artistes for the occasion.

Rustam Trifon was one of them. He was fifty-three. His poster was still pinned above Mimy's bed. He agreed to come to Impasse Tabouelle, and went up to her room, climbing the stairs with the grace of an angel. Then I asked him to pick a rose from the garden and he went and put it on Mimy's grave, in the Saint-Étienne cemetery. He looked very moved.

It was a sad and beautiful moment.

In the evening we stayed in the arena, Charles, Louise and I.

'Mimy would have loved it,' I said, looking at the huge velvet curtain beneath the rows of spotlights.

Charles and Louise didn't reply. Perhaps they thought Mimy could see everything from there. Hear everything, pick up the same emotions. Perhaps not. Since Mimy's death, they had rather lost sight of God.

We parted like that.

And I regretted, at the time, not mentioning my doubts.

The next day, Charles and Louise set off for the Île de Ré. The campsite where we used to go at Bois-Plage-en-Ré had been sold almost ten years before to make way for a new improved one. A luxury affair with a pool and tennis courts, where no child from Elbeuf would ever set foot. At about ten to seven in the evening, just before it closed, they went to the top of the lighthouse, the Phare des Baleines. Fifty-seven metres. Two hundred and fifty-seven steps. A cold wind was blowing from the Atlantic, they were on their own.

Hand in hand, they climbed the concrete balustrade and threw themselves into the void.

Afterwards, I often went to see Grandma Ninja on Route des Roches. She was the only survivor of my real family. We talked about it a lot. In the end I confessed what was weighing down my heart. She reassured me. I had been right not to say anything to Charles and Louise. It was better for them to have gone like that, convinced that Mimy had been murdered at random. With no one to accuse but fate. But she also gave me to understand that everything would gnaw away at me. That I had to get rid of it.

'How, Jeanine? How do I do that?'

'By telling the police everything. Even if it means reopening the worst old scars.'

And then I thought of that poem Mimy had written.

The last lines.

> *I will build a fortress around us*
> *And I will defend it*
> *M2O*

Mimy would never have been able to write that.

I missed Mimy so much.

31

Reopen the worst scars?

Mona switched off the ceiling light of the Fiat and turned to me.

'So?'

The brown envelope had fallen at my feet. I had trouble connecting everything I had just read with the murder of Morgane Avril, the suicide of Magali Verron, but plainly there was a link of some kind.

I just needed to unravel it all . . . The image of a red scarf tied too tightly around someone's neck came to mind.

Mona noticed that a tear was shining in the corner of my eyes.

'Moving?'

'Very.'

'About Morgane or Myrtille?'

'Myrtille. Mimy, rather . . . Such a charming declaration of love.'

Mona's eyes gleamed strangely. She hesitated, then put a delicate finger on my eyelid to wipe it.

'Thanks,' she said.

'For what?'

She didn't reply, just put the car into reverse and drove out of the garden.

At 11.10 p.m. Mona parked in Place Jean-Paul-Laurens, opposite Christian Le Medef's house. Not a cop in sight. Before crossing the car park, I pulled up the hood of my WindWall North Face. I stopped outside the fisherman's house.

'It wasn't locked yesterday.'

I turned the handle. The door opened.

'He's not suspicious, your witness!' Mona joked.

I waited until we were both inside, then shouted, 'Christian? Christian Le Medef?'

As I'd expected, there was no reply. Xanax, the former nuclear engineer, hadn't come home.

Escaped?

Kidnapped?

Murdered?

Mona followed me into the dark corridor, almost amused.

I stopped dead in my tracks. I felt cold, as if the temperature in the room had plummeted.

The staircase in front of us was in complete darkness.

'No light,' I whispered.

'Why would there be if there's no one home?'

'Yesterday, upstairs, the bedside light was on in Le Medef's bedroom.'

'You must have turned it off before you left.'

I shook my head. I was sure I hadn't touched it. With the tips of my fingers I turned on the torch app on my iPhone and shone it up the stairs.

Nothing. Not a sound. No sign of life. Just as it had been when I visited the previous evening.

Apart from the fact that the bedside light was out.

I climbed about ten steps to light up the landing, then stopped and called again.

'Le Medef?'

Nobody.

I was wrong again. I must have pressed the switch of that wretched lamp to turn it off without even noticing.

'Let's just see whether I'm mad or not!' I said to Mona as we went back down the stairs. 'Follow me.'

She let me go ahead of her along the corridor, and our bodies brushed against each other. The light from my mobile phone slid over the walls, illuminating the wallpaper which was coming away from the wall with the damp, the grey electric sockets, the rotting woodwork. Obsessed the previous day by the disappearance of Christian Le Medef, I hadn't noticed the extent to which the fisherman's house, which he was supposed to be maintaining, appeared to be almost abandoned.

I lowered the torch to light the black-and-white tiles. Only the sound of our footsteps on the floor disturbed the silence.

The silence . . .

Another shock ran through my body. Madness was stalking me, once again.

Someone had turned off the radio!

I murmured into the gloom, 'The radio was on yesterday.'

Mona didn't reply. I just felt her breath on my back. Shivers ran down my spine. What was I going to find in that room? I stopped in the doorway.

'Christian?'

Ridiculous. What was I thinking? That his kidnappers had brought him back during the day to finish his tagliatelle?

No answer, of course.

Who had called in after my visit? And why? To drop off Le Medef's corpse?

My torch swept the room towards the table in the middle, then the chair, the microwave, the television, the radio . . . Several times, in ever faster circles, almost hysterical after a few moments.

Like a lighting man who had lost his mind.

Then, throwing caution to the wind, I pressed the switch. The white light from a bare bulb exploded in the room, dazzling us. I held my hand over my eyes like a visor, unable to believe what I saw.

The room was empty.

Completely empty.

No chair, no table, no bottle, plate or glass, no television, not even a radio. And not even a single item of furniture.

The dining room and the kitchen had been cleared completely since the previous day.

Suddenly the phone in my hand weighed a ton. My head was spinning. Mona walked into the room. There was a faint echo as she did so.

'This is where Le Medef lived?'

'Yes.'

I overcame my feeling of dizziness and pointed one by one to the place where each piece of furniture had stood. I ran my fingers over the walls, over the floor. The traces of dust, or their absence, revealed that these objects had been moved recently. Everything had been taken away at great speed.

'They've completely cleared the place,' I said.

'Who are they?'

'I have no idea, Mona. But it wouldn't have been that difficult. A table, a chair, a few electrical items – you could get that all into a van . . .'

Mona said nothing. I carried on, thinking aloud:

'First they get rid of the awkward witness. Then all the other evidence—'

'A conspiracy? They're incredibly well organised, Jamal.'

There was a hint of irony in Mona's voice.

I turned towards her and took her by the shoulders.

'Damn it, Mona! Do you think I could have made it all up? Every detail? The glass of wine, the plate of tagliatelle, the radio on low? Do you think I'm that crazy?'

My words, too loud, bounced off the bare walls. Mona went and stood in the middle of the room, where Le Medef's chair had been the previous day.

'Let's stop asking ourselves that kind of question, Jamal. Let's just stick to the programme. You promised, remember? Tonight we were going to pay a surprise visit to your two witnesses. Christian Le Medef and Denise Joubain. Then you were going to hand yourself in.'

I didn't protest. I hadn't the strength.

We stayed in the house for a few more minutes, then Mona took me by the hand and led me out. As soon as we set foot in the street, the door of the house opposite opened. A faint light fell on the road. I instinctively stepped into the darkness. The man who came outside could only see Mona's outline.

'Not too warm, is it?'

A limping shadow slipped between his legs. I recognised the three-legged dog from last night. His master took an eternity to light a cigarette, long enough to take advantage of the light of the flame to assess Mona's face.

'It's not every night you see a pretty girl like you hanging about in the street.'

The three-legged dog limped towards me. Mona automatically called it over with a click of her tongue and crouched down to stroke it. The neighbour seemed to appreciate the gesture.

'Have you lived here for a long time?' she asked.

'Hmmm. Nearly ten years.' He took a drag on his cigarette. 'What were you doing in the house?'

This idiot had seen the light!

'Just visiting,' Mona replied, quite naturally.

I retreated further into the darkness, taking care to lift my left foot a few centimetres above the pavement.

'At this time of night?'

He looked amazed. With an instinctive reaction that surprised me, I gripped the butt of the King Cobra in my pocket. The man blew out some smoke and then shrugged.

'You'd think they'd do anything to sell . . .'

'To sell?' Mona asked.

'Yes. They've been looking for a buyer for six months. I'd have to say that Yport is hardly Deauville, you know? There are dozens of houses for sale like this one.'

My legs were shaking. I kept my balance by resting my hand on a cold piece of sandstone. Mona was playing innocent.

'So the house has been empty for six months?'

'Yeah. Apart from prospective buyers who come and look at it. But yes, that's pretty rare, particularly at this time of night.'

He spat out his cigarette butt and smiled at Mona, imagining, although he didn't really believe it, that she would make a charming neighbour, then he called his dog in. The door clicked shut behind him.

I waited, then walked through the darkness towards the Fiat. Mona's voice rang out behind me.

'Satisfied?'

I tried to come up with an explanation, but the best I could do was:

'An empty house! Ideal for setting someone up. You can move the furniture in and out, undisturbed.'

Mona turned on the lights of the Fiat.

'So Le Medef was an accomplice? I thought he was your ally? He was the one who gave you his address, isn't that right?'

'Perhaps he didn't trust me. He talked about a plot, about *omertà*. Perhaps he was frightened! Perhaps . . .'

Mona handed me the keys.

'OK, let's go, Jamal. I'll let you drive, seeing as how you know the way to Denise's house.'

Not another word.

She could have given me a thousand arguments to prove that I'd imagined the disappearance of Christian Le Medef. Then the removal of all his furniture. That the neighbour was the kind to notice a removal van parked outside his front door, for example. That basically the only witness I had to back me up, between last night and tonight, was a three-legged dog.

I started up the Fiat.

The instrument panel showed the time in fluorescent green figures: 11.32 p.m.

'Denise Joubain will have a heart attack at this time of night . . .'

'Or I will,' Mona said. 'What's the next surprise on the agenda? Denise with her throat ripped out by aliens? Her ghost offering us tea?

The ghost of Denise Joubain . . .

In the silence of the car, I remembered the old lady's words. She said she hadn't left her home for years. But she said she'd recognised me, she'd bumped into me before, but that was ten years ago, on the beach at Yport, on the morning of Morgane Avril's murder. My last hope rested on the testimony of a senile old woman whose ravings would only help to convince me of my own amnesia.

*

252

Sitting in the passenger seat, Mona had turned on the roof light and was flicking through the files of Morgane Avril and Magali Verron that I had stolen from Carmen Avril and Piroz. Concentrating. I suddenly had a sense that she had read something that disturbed her. Her eyes kept darting from one file to the other.

I slowed down as we turned into the long straight road leading to the old railway station of Tourville-les-Ifs.

'Have you found something?'

She gave me a strange look.

It was obvious.

She had found something. Something that had upset her.

'No. Maybe.'

'What?'

'Not now. After the old lady.'

'Why?'

Mona's tone changed abruptly.

'After the old lady, damn it.'

32

Did you find something?

The Fiat's headlights lit up the Orient Express carriage, then the Pacific Chapelon locomotive, and finally the façade of the former station, whose clock still stood at 7.34.

As soon as I'd turned off the engine, the station, the trains and the car park disappeared into darkness. We walked by the light of our torches. The two beams passed along the pastel-blue walls of the station-master's house.

'Shall we wake Denise?' Mona asked.

Before replying, I clutched the door handle. Closed, this time. The hamlet of Les Ifs consisted only of a few detached houses whose silhouettes could just be seen about fifty metres away.

'We're going to wake up the whole neighbourhood if we hammer on the door.'

Without even taking time to think, I walked towards the lattice window. The shutters weren't closed. I picked up a stone the size of an egg and knocked it sharply against the pane closest to the handle. Ten centimetres by ten. A brief cascade of broken glass tinkled in the silence. Without taking any additional precautions, I opened the window from inside.

Some drops of blood trickled along my palm. Shallow cuts. Mona looked at me without a word.

'We'll give Denise a nice surprise,' I joked.

The tone wasn't quite right.

Why break in? To battle against the evidence they were piling up against me? What did I expect? To surprise an army of conspirators at Denise Joubain's house, busy constructing a new stage set, erecting a new chamber of illusions?

We climbed in through the window.

Arnold, I thought. *Arnold will spot us!*

Strangely, there was no sign of the shih-tzu. I tried to remember the arrangement of the rooms of the old railway station. Denise's bedroom was diagonally opposite.

My torch lit up the walls.

I felt a huge sense of relief. Reassuring, almost burning warmth. The photographs of trains were still on the walls! The Orient Express crossed Venice Lagoon, the Shinkansen slipped into its Japanese city. My torch went on inspecting the room, sliding over the exposed beams, the dresser, the dried flowers in the vase, the wicker chairs.

Every detail was as I remembered! A few neurones in my brain were still making connections. For the first time in ages I could trust my memory. I hadn't dreamed that demented discussion with Denise.

I hesitated between calling Denise Joubain's name, as I had done for Christian Le Medef, surprising her in her bed to give her a heart attack, shaking her, putting her under the shower, torturing her until she remembered our meeting on the beach at Yport on Wednesday, with Piroz and the corpse of Magali Verron.

We approached the bedroom. As I pushed the door, the trainer screwed on to the prosthesis of my left foot touched a soft object on the floor.

A surreal squeak ripped through the silence. A plastic squeaky toy. A giraffe.

Almost immediately the light came on in Denise Joubain's bedroom. My retinas exploded. I gripped the revolver in my pocket. Don't let the old woman scream. Don't give her time to raise the alarm this time. Don't . . .

The walls of the old woman's bedroom were covered with Hello Kitty wallpaper.

Fairies dangled above my head from a wire on the ceiling. Elves climbed along the curtain. Giant soft toys were piled up. Dogs, rabbits and elephants. More fairies whirled above the turquoise bed. Inside it, two dazzled eyes stared at me. A child of about six.

A cry made me turn my head. It came from a second, smaller bed on my right, this one with pink stripes.

The head of a little girl of about three appeared. Terrified. The child screamed without interruption, without even breathing, without worrying about the fact that her cheeks, her forehead were turning bright red.

'Christ, Jamal.'

Mona seemed incapable of uttering another word. As if until now she had been understanding about the crazy trail I was pursuing, but this time I had crossed the line.

I turned on my heel, trying to find some way to reassure the little girl.

Waste of time.

The boy was now shouting even louder than his sister, his thin body curled up in his pirate pyjamas.

'What the hell are you doing here?' a voice thundered behind us.

We turned to see a woman in a nightdress, pale, mute with horror. The speaker, a bare-chested man in his forties, with grey hair, was brandishing a kitchen knife in his right hand.

Mona's damp palm settled on my shoulder as I turned the King Cobra on the two parents.

A reflex action, without thinking.

The children's cries grew louder than ever. The mother, like a she-wolf, seemed to be poised to throw herself on these two strangers who were separating her from her children.

Mona's voice was pleading:

'Jamal, no.'

I gripped the butt of the revolver.

'What are you doing here?' I demanded.

'What?'

The father, though taken aback, held my eye. He didn't show the slightest sign of fear.

I said it again: 'What are you doing here?'

He didn't seem to understand the meaning of my question, but he answered anyway.

'We've rented the cottage for the week . . .'

Mona sighed and tugged my sleeve.

'It's OK, Jamal. Let's go . . .'

I didn't move. The King Cobra was only a replica, but the man with the knife didn't know that.

'And yesterday?' I asked. 'Were you here early yesterday afternoon?'

'No,' said the father. 'We spent the whole day at the D-Day beaches, but . . .'

His voice gained in confidence the more questions I asked. Perhaps he thought he was dealing with some crazy police officers . . .

Mona pulled my arm again.

'Come on. You're scaring me.'

I followed her, slowly, keeping the gun pointed at the parents. The mother dashed towards her little girl, who fell silent as if by magic. The father didn't take his eyes off us, and still held the knife pointed in our direction.

Mona's hand grabbed mine, urging me to beat a hasty retreat. The knick-knacks from the old railway station danced a sarabande in my head. The trains on the walls, the wicker chairs, the fairies on the ceiling.

Bloody hell, I couldn't have invented all those details! I had a perfectly clear memory of those photographs, that furniture, the position of every object in that room.

As soon as we had passed through the door of the old railway station, Mona forced me to run. I remembered that, a few hours earlier, Arnold had run after me into the car park, as if he had always lived here and was defending his territory with all his doggy fury. Two children's bicycles, one with stabilisers and one without, leaned against the wall. An Audi with a Paris registration was parked a few metres further away.

Mona drove this time, without a word. I kept up a monologue, as if trying to convince myself, firing out frantic arguments until I ran out of ideas.

'So the former station is a holiday cottage, fine. The family has hired it for the week, OK. But they left it empty all day yesterday. There would have been time to tidy the kids' toys away in the bedroom, so Denise could move in and play out that part for me. Tell me the story of her railwayman husband. Claim not to remember Magali Verron's suicide.'

Mona didn't reply. We hadn't driven three hundred metres before she turned abruptly to the right and stopped the car in a huge deserted car park, in front of a long concrete building.

'Entrepôt Bénédictine', it said in big red letters. Benedictine Warehouse. The place looked abandoned.

Mona turned off the engine.

'This is the end of the road, Jamal. I've gone as far as I can.'

'Listen to me, Mona . . .'

In my mind's eye I saw the framed photographs of trains. The Magistral Baikal-Amur stuck in the snow, the slopes of the Andes and the dykes crossing the sea. The pictures I'd seen the day before in the old railway station of Les Ifs.

'Jamal, it's over. Denise Joubain has never lived in that railway station. Any more than Christian Le Medef lived in that house on Place Jean-Paul-Larens. You never spoke to them, they never saw that girl jumping off the cliff. They didn't, and neither did anyone else. No journalist. No police officer. Because Magali Verron has never existed, Jamal. You made her up. I don't know why, but you created that girl out of nothing. It probably has something to do with Morgane Avril, because you gave her the same face. And perhaps with the murder of Myrtille Camus. That's probably why the police are after you, but one thing is certain, Jamal, and it's actually good news. The police can't pin the rape and murder of Magali Verron on you: the girl doesn't exist.'

I picked up the police file, the one I stole from Piroz.

MAGALI VERRON, written in capital letters.

'I couldn't have invent—'

With an exasperated wave of her hand, Mona gestured to me to be quiet.

'We've had that conversation already. I've fulfilled my part of the bargain, Jamal. It's up to you to fulfil yours. You'll hand yourself over to the police as soon as the sun rises.'

I refused to give in.

'Damn it, Mona, that's what they're waiting for! OK, for the moment, we're getting nowhere, but there are still other possibilities to explore, don't you think? This business about the prisoner's dilemma, for example. And the mail I've been getting! I'm not crazy enough to leave those envelopes lying in the glove compartment and forget.'

Mona looked at me affectionately in a way that reminded me of the shrinks at the Saint Antoine Institute when they were listening to the fanciful explanations of young people caught lying.

Fuck it! I wasn't giving up.

'The explanation is in these letters! Something that no one's noticed, Mona. And I'm the only one who can find it . . .'

She ran her hand tenderly through my hair. A gesture more maternal than passionate.

'Forget it, Jamal. Forget the present. Forget everything that's happened over the last three days. You've imagined the whole thing.' Her forefinger came down to my forehead. 'You've imagined it because the truth is in your head somewhere, buried deep. You need to look for what happened ten years ago rather than what happened this week.'

Without thinking, I grabbed her wrist and clutched it tightly, too tightly, before throwing it on her lap like a dead branch.

My voice was icy.

'You too, then.'

'You too what?'

'You're playing this little game as well. Driving me mad to make me the scapegoat! Pin the murders of those two girls ten years ago on me. That's the goal, isn't it? Make me crack? Make me confess?'

I thought again of the envelopes in the glove compartment of the

Fiat 500, of the postman delivering mail to Vaucottes. Whoever was responsible had to have set up those deliveries in advance, anticipating my every move. Only Mona could have organised all this. She was part of this conspiracy.

'That's it, Mona. From here on I'm going it alone.'

She tried to rest her hand on mine. I brushed it away.

'I don't trust you any more, Mona. I don't trust anyone any more.'

I realised that I was a total bastard.

Maybe . . .

Mona had taken incredible risks for me.

Or not.

To give her the benefit of the doubt would have meant taking a risk. A risk I could no longer afford. I was going to get up, leave the Fiat and disappear into the night. Mona opened the door.

'Keep the car, Jamal. You're going to need it more than I do . . .'

Again her gaze shifted from the Magali Verron file to Morgane Avril's. I remembered that she'd discovered something before we parked in front of the old railway station, something that had convinced her that I was raving.

Not now. After the old lady, she had said.

Too late to ask her.

She stepped outside, then leaned back in. Illuminated by the street lamp a few metres away. The playful expression had been replaced by the look of a hunted animal that wouldn't live to see another year. Tears ran down her cheeks.

'There's one more thing, Jamal. There's still a piece missing from your puzzle. Something important that you've overlooked.'

She was crying even harder now.

An important fact that I'd overlooked?

I was trying to work out what she meant, when Mona spelled it out for me:

'You've fallen in love with this girl, Jamal. With Morgane Avril. With that face you've described to me so many times. So noble, so pure, so sad. That face you thought you saw again three days ago at the top of the cliff. Before it slipped through your fingers

260

and disappeared over the cliff. You're fantasising about a corpse, my love! A pretty little dead corpse, buried ten years ago. Sorry, I'm no match for that. I can't be jealous of a ghost.'

'The girl exists, Mona.'

She smiled at me without answering, then walked in front of the Fiat. She studied the straight, empty road for a long time and then took an object from her jacket.

A flash of gold sparkled in the night.

'You can have this back,' Mona said.

She set the sheriff's star down on the bonnet of the car.

I couldn't speak.

'Good luck,' she whispered through the open door.

The sheriff's star. The five peaks I had to climb . . .

The five directions of my star, like everything else, had been swept away by the torment of the last few days. Curiously, they ran through my head as Mona walked away, swallowed by the darkness of the car park. *Become, Make, Have, Be, Pay.*

Lost in my thoughts, it took me a while to notice that Mona had turned around. Then, as she approached the Fiat again, I thought she was going to come back to me, kiss me, hold me in her arms, collapse in tears and ask my forgiveness.

She merely lifted the windscreen wiper.

What was she playing at, damn it?

Slowly, with one finger, she wrote in the dust of the windscreen. Twelve letters.

MAGALI VERRON

Then her finger started erasing a letter, just one, then writing the same letter a few centimetres below.

M first.

Then O.

Then R.

Then G.

Then all the rest.

When each of the twelve letters had been erased and written on another line a few centimetres lower but in a different order, a new name appeared in the dust of the windscreen.

MORGANE AVRIL

Mona leaned towards the door of the Fiat 500 again.

'One and the same woman, Jamal. A dead woman and her ghost . . .'

At the end of the road two headlights flashed and then, almost immediately, the glare from a revolving light pierced the night with a blue whirl.

33

A dead woman and her ghost?

The police van suddenly changed course to climb the embankment and come to rest a few metres from the Fiat 500.

Full beam. Two suns shining straight ahead, while an electric-blue sky spun around.

For a moment I wondered how the police had been able to find us so easily. Just for a moment.

What an idiot!

Obviously, as soon as we left, the couple from the old railway station cottage had called the police. A guy with a gun had broken into their house, they'd found him standing in their children's room.

An Arab. Crippled. Excited.

And obviously the cavalry had charged.

Two shadows emerged from the van. I recognised Piroz's heavy silhouette, and the long, bent-backed outline of his deputy.

The captain's voice called into the night.

'Salaoui, game's up. Get out of the car with your hands in the air.'

Piroz and his deputy were each holding a gun. They came forward by a metre. The headlights behind them made them look vast. Mona recoiled until she was pressed against the bonnet of the Fiat, as if frightened by the disproportionate size of their weapons.

Piroz shouted again.

'Don't move, Mademoiselle Salinas.'

I was frozen in the car, unable to take the slightest decision. I felt

263

the weight of the King Cobra in my pocket. A pathetic weapon that only fired rubber bullets.

'Out of the car now, Salaoui!'

I opened the door. Calmly.

I felt what one must feel before dying: intense resignation, but at the same time the ultimate excitement . . . Knowing at last what lies hidden behind it all. The explanation of the great mystery.

Who was I?

An amnesiac madman or a trapped scapegoat?

'Step forward, Salaoui!'

My eyes swept the car park of the Benedictine warehouse. Less than ten metres away, the tarmac was engulfed in darkness.

'Don't try anything,' Piroz barked again, 'I don't want to shoot you.'

I only had to sprint to lose myself in the darkness, a simple thrust of the hips should do it. Would the police really fire?

'Do as they say,' Mona pleaded.

As I got to my feet I pressed my left hand against the car, in the shadow of the bodywork. I felt Mona's warmth less than a metre away, her crazed breathing. I took my decision in a second.

The worst one possible.

Try my luck. Push it as far as it would go.

The reflex of a street urchin, like any kid from the estates at the sight of a uniform. *Run!*

Slowly, I raised my right hand while my left hand, hidden against the door, rummaged in the pocket of my WindWall.

Then it all happened very quickly.

I suddenly raised my left arm, my hand gripping the King Cobra, aiming for the stars, so that Piroz was surprised by two contradictory pieces of information.

Simultaneously.

I was armed. I was giving myself up.

I figured I could take advantage of that moment's hesitation to jump into the night, run due east, first cover the thirty metres of car park, then the kilometres of flat fields. My hundreds of hours of training would save my skin.

The shot rang out without warning.

Piroz had fired at me. Point-blank.

No pain.

Simultaneously, Piroz and his deputy lowered their guns, silent with dread.

As if in slow motion, Mona slumped on top of me.

The King Cobra danced frantically in my fist, while Mona's body shuddered against my shoulder. Blood spilled from her chest, drenching her swamp-green jumper. A second scarlet thread trickled from her lips.

My heart was pounding till I thought it would break.

Anger. Fear. Hatred.

Mona was suffocating. Inaudible words escaped from her throat, mute mysteries murmured in angels' ears. Her eyes gently darkened, as if discovering a landscape that no one had ever looked upon, then they went out.

For ever.

Mona's body slipped against mine until it fell, face down on the tarmac, almost without a sound, with the elegance of a ballerina dying on stage.

My trembling hands tried to control the King Cobra. In the gloom it was impossible to tell the make of the revolver that I was aiming at them. I tried my luck.

Barrel of the gun aimed straight at Piroz's face.

Slowly, I walked around the Fiat to sit down on the driver's side. The two cops, arms dangling, didn't move an inch, as if crushed by the weight of their blunder.

One certainty stabbed at my heart.

The cops hadn't given me a chance! They had shot to kill. Mona had been in the firing line; she was dead because she didn't believe me.

I had been right all along.

The cops were trying to trap me. Whatever the consequences.

I glanced one last time at Mona lying on the tarmac, then put all the weight of my grief on the accelerator.

The sound of metal rang out in the silence. Gold dust sparkled on the bonnet of the Fiat.

My guts twisted. Foot to the floor.

The sheriff's star balanced there for a moment, then toppled into the car park. In films, the heroine wears it on her heart, and the bullet bounces off it. She doesn't die . . .

In films.

The Fiat leapt. I heard the front right tyre driving over the gilded iron insignia that my mother had bought for five francs. It was another time. The time my mother had dreamed for me, when I would arrest the bad guys.

The Benedictine warehouses whizzed by, endlessly. I aimed between two hedges to get back to the main road. Dark and deserted.

On the way to hell. I wouldn't see Mona again.

But the ghost of Morgane Avril . . . perhaps.

34

In another life?

I drove for another few moments along the forest path, then stopped the Fiat 500. As I turned the ignition key I had the feeling that I was breaking up the universe all around me, cutting off with a single motion all forms of civilised life. The headlights, the luminous signs on the dashboard, but also the stars and the moon, invisible behind the arch of the trees. Pitch darkness.

I stayed like that for a long time, in total blackness.

Then I opened the door, leaned out and vomited on to the grass and over the tyre of Mona's car. Once I was done, I pressed my back and my neck against the driver's seat. I stayed that way for several minutes, unmoving. Tears ran down my cheeks, and I didn't make the slightest effort to wipe them away. They ran down to my lips, mingling with the bitter taste in my throat. For a moment I imagined that the visions produced by my raving brain might spill out like vomit, flood from my lachrymal glands like tears. Flow out in my blood too, were I to slit a vein.

The smell and the taste were becoming unbearable. My hand reached out to turn on the roof light.

Twelve letters appeared, as if etched on the dirty windscreen.

MORGANE AVRIL

In my mind I saw Mona's silhouette writing them with her finger, her weary smile, her last words as she left my star on the bonnet.

Good luck.

What did luck care about us, Mona?

A thin fog rose over the undergrowth, as if smoke were coming out of the ground. The thermometer of the Fiat showed that it was minus two.

Soon the twelve letters disappeared in a cocoon of fog.

An illusion.

I had to accept it. Magali Verron had never existed. Nor anything that might have been connected with her death.

No witness, scarf, rape or murder by strangling.

An anagram. A ghost. A fantasy.

I jumped from one thought to the next as if they were stepping stones.

If none of it was true, why had Piroz been hunting me down for three days? And why did he have no hesitation about shooting me?

Another stone. This one was moving unsteadily beneath me.

If nothing was true about Magali Verron's suicide, when had I first seen Piroz? Not on the beach at Yport beach that morning, with his deputy. Had I met him for the first time at Fécamp police station, the day when I first met Mona? So the police had called me in for a completely different reason. Another case. And I'd made up this whole story.

Another jump. Another stone. The far bank was barely visible in the distance.

Something didn't add up! The French police don't shoot at suspects! Not without warning. Not point-blank. Not to kill. I had aimed the King Cobra at the sky. I had never threatened Piroz. But he had fired to keep me from getting away. He would rather have shot me down than let me run away. Why?

Because he was sure that I was the rapist who had murdered Morgane Avril and Myrtille Camus, a serial killer that the police had been after for ten years? Because, even if I had forgotten everything, they had accumulated enough evidence to be certain of my guilt?

My fingers touched the icy windscreen. The twelve invisible letters taunted me, impossible to erase.

I had heard the shrinks talking about such things at the Saint Antoine Institute. Kids denying atrocities they had been subjected to. No, their parents weren't rapists. No, they hadn't been molested. Yes, they wanted to go back home. Those kids manufactured a different life for themselves, one that was easier to bear. In their heads at least.

The fog engulfed the Fiat, making it look as if it was floating silently through the clouds.

Was that what had happened in my case? Except I wasn't a child who had been raped. I wasn't a traumatised victim.

I was a monster.

I had killed those girls ten years before.

I, and I alone, was responsible for Mona's death.

I went into the forest. The cold gripped me like a vice around my chest. I didn't care. Icy puddles cracked beneath my feet. I walked unsteadily for several metres. I lost my balance on a thick patch of black ice. My hands gripped the trunk of the nearest tree, an elm whose bark tore my palms.

Then I yelled into the silence.

No!!!

Some leaves trembled ten metres in front of me. A rabbit, a bird, some animal that I had startled. Do woodland creatures have nightmares? Are they only afraid of the night?

Desperate to escape, I yelled again.

No!!!

I kept my cry going for an eternity, not even breathing, until my eardrums felt as if they would burst. One final barrier in my brain refused to yield.

No, I repeated at last.

Almost a murmur this time.

No.

I didn't remember murdering Morgane Avril and Myrtille Camus. I didn't remember for one simple reason.

I was innocent!

Three days ago I had watched as Magali Verron threw herself off a cliff. I stood over her body on the beach with Christian Le Medef and Denise Joubain. There was a key that explained everything, very close by, within reach. A detail that I had to decode, like the prisoner's dilemma, or that poem Myrtille Camus had sent to her fiancé, signed M2O.

I wiped my palms against my jeans to get rid of the drops of blood that were forming on them. The mixture of bile and tears in my mouth made me feel nauseous. I couldn't collapse, die there in the cold, wait for the police to come and pick up a guy who had been eaten up by remorse. A beast at the end of his tether, who would be finished off without being questioned any further. I remembered Mona's last act of kindness at Martin Denain's, in Vaucottes. Coffee and biscuits.

I walked to the boot of the Fiat, running through the events of the last three days in my head once more.

The events of the last few days could not have happened by chance. They followed a preordained pattern, there was a logic . . .

The dew settling on the car was already turning into a fine layer of ice.

. . . but it wasn't the kind of logic improvised in the heat of the moment, linking a series of steps the way a reader strings together the chapters of a detective thriller. I had to take a step back, take stock, on my own. Stop, sleep.

Or drink a litre of coffee.

I opened the boot.

Like an ice sculpture, I stood frozen beside the Fiat, unable to move.

Beside the thermos and the packet of biscuits was a brown envelope.

Addressed to me.

Who but a ghost could have put it there?

Who but me?

I took the time to eat the biscuits, Lotus-brand Speculoos from Martin Denain's larder, and drink two cups of hot coffee, strong, no sugar.

Then I opened the envelope.

35

Something didn't add up?

Avril–Camus case – spring 2007

The regional crime squad were officially taken off the Avril–Camus investigation on 9 June 2007. Commander Léo Bastinet hadn't come up with any new leads in almost a year and no one had looked at any of the three thousand pages of the case file. Judge Paul-Hugo Lagarde, with Léo Bastinet's agreement, suggested passing the management of the Avril–Camus file to the Fécamp brigade until the statute of limitations ran out.

The Fécamp police had been the first to investigate the murder, they had remained involved in the investigation, and Captain Grima, who had been sidelined after the second murder, would probably see it as a small personal revenge when the case came back to him, after all the efforts of the regional crime squad had come to nothing.

Captain Grima accepted the case, and the files of the double investigation were transferred from Caen to Fécamp on Friday, 15 June 2007. The next day he received a visit from Carmen Avril. She came back a few days later, and then almost every week during the summer. Then Grima worked out that Judge Lagarde hadn't just given him a case that had reached a dead end, he had lumbered him with a pain in the neck who had been hassling the legal system and the police for years.

Never forget.

Time had done nothing to diminish the determination of the president of the Fil Rouge Association, who was now in sole charge since the double suicide of Charles and Louise Camus.

Three years later, Grima received his transfer to the police in Saint-Florent, a small port town in Corsica, wedged between Cap Corse and the Agriates desert. Perhaps he had grown weary of the assaults of the waves that crashed against the sea wall of Fécamp, or perhaps it was the assaults of Carmen Avril that drove him away. The police captain and the proprietor of the Dos-d'Âne had never got on. Before leaving, Grima handed the keys of the case to the oldest officer in the station, an experienced detective who had been responsible for interviewing the witnesses who'd encountered the stranger with the red scarf: Sonia Thurau, the cloakroom girl, Mickey the bouncer, Vincent Carré, the chemistry student.

Captain Piroz.

A methodical worker, and one that Carmen Avril actually liked. Piroz had immediately agreed with her: they should be looking for a stranger who had been in Yport and Isigny on the dates when the murders occurred. He was not alarmed by the prospect of having to sift through lists of several thousand individuals to find the one name common to both lists. On the contrary, Piroz had a tenacity bordering on obsession. An old bachelor. No children. No talent or liking for football, detective novels or dominoes. He spent his evenings going through the case the way others might build models of the Benedictine Palace out of matchsticks.

All for nothing . . .

Piroz came no closer to the identity of the killer than Captain Grima, Commander Bastinet or criminal psychologist Ellen Nilsson.

After the death of Louise and Charles Camus, Carmen Avril held the reins of the Fil Rouge Association, even though it now had no reason to exist but a duty of memory celebrated every year at a gloomy AGM.

Carmen Avril, mother of Morgane Avril, president
Frédéric Saint-Michel, fiancé of Myrtille Camus, vice president
Océane Avril, sister of Morgane Avril, secretary
Jeanine Dubois, grandmother of Myrtille Camus, deputy secretary
Alina Masson, best friend of Myrtille Camus, treasurer

The rare meetings of the association were an opportunity for Alina to get closer to Océane. They had both lost a twin sister, whether the tie was emotional or one of blood. Amputated from the other half of themselves. They got on, even though Océane had inherited from her mother, and probably from the rape of her sister, a stubborn hatred of men that she struggled to contain during their long nocturnal conversations. For the first time Alina opened up and dared to expose the doubts that had eaten away at her for years. Océane listened to her and didn't talk to anybody, not even her mother, then advised Alina to resume contact with the police who had investigated Myrtille's murder. With Ellen Nilsson rather than Bastinet. The criminal psychologist knew the file as well as the commander did, but would be more likely to understand. Perhaps.

Ellen Nilsson refused to talk to Alina Masson. The Avril–Camus file had been closed for four years, and she claimed to have other more pressing cases to deal with.

Ten phone calls didn't change anything.

They would have to go through Piroz, who in turn put pressure on Judge Lagarde to make the criminal psychologist agree to see the police captain and Myrtille Camus's best friend at her Paris office on Rue d'Aubigné. Piroz growled his way through a journey on the dirty, stinking metro, nearly got knocked over at Place de la Concorde, cursed again as he crammed his belly into the wrought-iron lift that went up to Nilsson's office on the fourth floor, south facing, with a view of the Seine.

Alina said nothing.

When Ellen herself opened the heavy oak door, wearing a Ralph Lauren dress that revealed her brand-new cleavage, she almost turned and left.

Likely to understand?

Piroz, visibly impressed by the customised curves, stood blocking her retreat.

They took a seat. Leather armchairs. Low glass table. Panoramic view of the Île Saint-Louis and the constant ballet of the *bateaux-mouches*. Alina felt suddenly dizzy. How could she progress towards the truth without damaging the memory of Myrtille?

Ellen crossed her perfect legs and wrinkled her smooth forehead into the best frown that she could muster.

'You wanted to see me, Mademoiselle Masson?'

Alina had no choice but to dive in.

'You remember,' she managed to say at length, 'the first time we met at the regional crime squad in Caen, just after Myrtille's murder. You asked a question. One that took me by surprise.'

'Which one was that?' said Ellen, who clearly hadn't reviewed the notes on their meeting six years ago.

'You asked why Myrtille was wearing such a sexy outfit on the day she was raped. A short, sky-blue dress with hibiscus flowers. Matching mauve underwear. Not the usual outfit for a camp activity leader.'

'That's possible. We pursued so many theories . . .'

'What were you thinking at that moment?' Alina pressed.

Ellen delved into her memory, then replied wearily:

'Nothing specific. If I remember correctly, Bastinet thought we should be focusing on potential culprits, not the victims. Basically he was right, both Myrtille Camus and Morgane Avril were victims chosen at random.'

Piroz yawned.

'I've thought a lot about that question over the years,' Alina went on. 'To tell the truth, I've never stopped thinking about it. You were right: Myrtille didn't usually dress like that.'

'But Myrtille died on her day off! As I recall, that's what you told me at the time.'

'Even on a day off, Myrtille wouldn't have dressed like that.'

Ellen's frown deepened.

'What do you mean, Mademoiselle Masson? Are you suggesting

that she knew her rapist? That . . . that she had arranged to meet him, is that it?'

Alina hesitated. Hanging on the wall, in a glass frame, was a huge photograph of a naked woman on her knees, her face hidden by a cascade of blonde hair.

Ellen?

It was plainly supposed to look that way.

'Yes,' Alina said at last. 'Myrtille had arranged to meet someone. A man. Probably her murderer.'

'Wasn't she engaged to that guy who played the guitar?'

Alina's face turned pink. She had said nothing during all those years for one reason. To protect Myrtille. Not to tarnish the image that her family kept of her. Perfect. Faithful. Loving.

'Yes . . .'

'Chichin, something like that?'

'Chichin was his nickname. His name is Frédéric Saint-Michel.'

For the first time the criminal psychologist leaned over the file on the low table in front of her. She flicked through a few pages and then looked up.

'So Myrtille was the victim of a womaniser, something like that? A charmer who had turned her head? You know, Mademoiselle Masson, your belief corresponds precisely to Captain Grima's original theory. Morgane Avril wasn't the victim of a stalker who came out of nowhere, but a seducer who lured her.'

Alina nodded and didn't say a word. Of course, she knew . . .

'Which changes nothing,' Ellen Nilsson went on. 'Charmer or predator, how does that get us any closer to identifying the murderer? Unless, of course, we know who Myrtille had arranged to meet. Do you have any idea, Mademoiselle Masson?'

'No.'

'Could it have been Olivier Roy, the guy with the Adidas cap who was prowling around her at the camp in Isigny? The one who disappeared a few months after the murder?'

For the first time, Piroz spoke. Ellen, surprised, turned towards the police captain.

'Impossible! Olivier Roy had a cast-iron alibi for the evening of

Morgane Avril's murder. And his DNA doesn't correspond to that of the rapist.'

'Exactly,' the criminal psychologist concluded. 'That was why poor Bastinet's investigation ran aground. An appointment with whom, then?'

'I don't know,' Alina said.

Tears glittered in the corners of her eyes, and she took a paper handkerchief from her pocket. Ellen bent over the file for a long time. Piroz took advantage of the fact to twist his neck around and compare the breasts of the blonde displayed on the wall with the ones he could make out beneath the psychologist's forget-me-not dress. When she straightened up, Piroz abruptly diverted his gaze towards the *bateaux-mouches*. A child caught in the act. Ellen's eyes, on the other hand, moved towards the photograph and stopped there as if before a mirror, then she flicked away a piece of invisible dust that had fallen between her breasts.

'I have to admit,' she went on, 'that even after all these years, some details are still disturbing. The sexy dress that Myrtille didn't usually wear, for example. The blue Moleskine notebook that was never found, when everyone stated that Myrtille recorded her most secret thoughts in it, and perhaps even the identity of the man she had arranged to meet. This Olivier Roy, of whom there is still no sign in spite of the posters with his face distributed all over the region, who disappeared for ever as soon as the police net began to close in on him. And the little pair of panties, too.'

Alina gave a start.

'What little pair of panties?'

The criminal psychologist turned first to Piroz and then to Alina.

'A detail. Of course, I assumed you were aware. No semen was found in Myrtille's vagina, but there were traces on her panties, which were found about a hundred metres away, in the channel of the Baie des Veys.'

No, Alina wasn't aware of it. Piroz probably was, but he was distracted once again by the indecent prayer of the girl behind the glass.

'Did the forensic experts have an explanation for that?' Alina wanted to know.

'The rapist must have intended to withdraw before orgasm, but he only managed to do so partially, and ejaculated on Myrtille, or at least on her panties. So we asked ourselves, why would he have wanted to withdraw? Was it because his sperm might get him into trouble?'

'Because,' Alina suggested, 'his DNA was registered on the police database in connection with another crime?'

'Except that it wasn't.'

Piroz lowered his eyes and spoke:

'Perhaps the rapist hoped that Myrtille Camus's murder wouldn't be linked with the killing of Morgane Avril.'

'Hardly likely,' Ellen replied. 'It would have been difficult not to make the connection between the two crimes, even if the rapist's DNA hadn't been a match. Two girls raped, strangled, in the same region, with the same scarf . . .'

Piroz grumbled. 'We're dealing with a deranged mind here . . .'

'Or,' Alina said tonelessly, 'there's a third possibility. Could it mean that he knew Myrtille, that he anticipated police would want to test his DNA?'

Ellen Nilsson let a second pass before replying.

'That's what we thought at first. We took the DNA of over one and a half thousand individuals – the family of Myrtille Camus, her friends, the inhabitants of Isigny, Elbeuf and the surrounding area. Every single person who might have been close to her. None of them were a match!'

Alina remained silent.

Why would the rapist have wanted to conceal his DNA, a voice repeated in her head, if he didn't know Myrtille? Did he know Morgane Avril? Everything was getting muddled. The torn dress with the hibiscus flowers, Olivier Roy prowling around her best friend on the beach and off the Îles Saint-Marcouf, the sky-blue Moleskine notebook, that poem sent to Fredéric, crutches and jonquils, caterpillars and fortresses, signed M2O. Marriage 2 October . . .

'And what about your search for the stranger who was in both places?' Ellen asked. 'Is that getting anywhere?'

Alina, lost in her thoughts, didn't reply.

'Slowly,' Piroz admitted. 'We're in no hurry. We have our whole lives—'

'Not entirely,' Ellen corrected him. 'You know as well as I do, after ten years without any fresh evidence the case is closed. The rapist will have won.'

'Well?' Alina asked in the lift.

She pressed herself against the wrought iron to avoid contact with Piroz's body.

'So,' she said again. 'What do you think?'

'It's not her,' Piroz said.

'What do you mean, it isn't her?'

'It isn't her in the picture! The pretty naked blonde, it's not the shrink. She's messing with us.'

A little later, in the metro, between Bastille and Saint-Paul, Piroz, jostled by a group of seven-year-old children all wearing the same caps, who had just invaded the carriage, pressed himself against Alina. This time she couldn't avoid it. He whispered in her ear:

'I saw that little smile on your lips earlier when she asked about the search for the stranger. You might think it's a waste of time, but the one thing we can be certain of is that the killer was in Yport on 5 June 2004 and in Isigny three months later.'

The children were yelling and Alina had to raise her voice.

'But there were thousands of people passing through. And the killer could have arrived by car or even on foot, without anyone seeing him arrive or leave – without his name appearing anywhere.'

Louvre.

Piroz shrugged. His eye wandered to a poster advertising Dior. Charlize Theron's naked silhouette reminded him of the one on the shrink's wall.

'I know,' he admitted. 'But pursuing that connection is stopping Carmen and her daughter Océane from going mad. Waiting and hoping, that's all they have left.'

Concorde.

The kids with the caps, ushered by two teachers, disappeared faster than a flock of pigeons. Alina took a step back and maintained a metre's distance between herself and the captain.

'Wait for what?' she asked. 'For the rapist to start again?'

Six years had passed since Myrtille's murder.

'Too late,' Piroz replied. 'He won't start again.'

Champs-Élysées-Clemenceau.

More Charlize Therons passed by. Four metres by three. Dior was bludgeoning people's minds, and Piroz loved it. Alina pursed her lips. Is this how impulses come into being? she wondered.

'He won't start again,' Piroz repeated, absorbed by a patch of white skin enlarged a thousand times.

Alina thought otherwise.

36

Is this how impulses come into being?

I crossed the Seine by the Pont de Brotonne at about one in the morning. Then I switched between motorways and secondary roads. The names of the Norman villages that I systematically avoided passed by on signposts illuminated by the Fiat's headlights. Pont-Audemer. Beuzeville. Pont-l'Évêque.

The pages that I had just read scrolled through my head. The identity of the red-scarf killer had to be buried somewhere in the details relating to the murder of Myrtille Camus. That information hadn't been given to me for no reason. That proof of my innocence was there, within reach.

An illusion? One more illusion?

Would it make any more sense after my final, headlong flight to Isigny-sur-Mer?

My phone rang in the depths of my pocket just before the turn-off for Troarn. It was almost two in the morning.

Piroz, of course . . .

I didn't pick up. Piroz had inherited the Avril–Camus case, they had been careful to let me know that by giving me that envelope. After all those years, that monomaniacal cop had finally found his culprit.

Me!

A few seconds later, a pinging noise indicated that someone had left a message. Still driving, I picked up the phone.

I almost let go of the wheel with surprise.

I was completely wrong!

It wasn't that bastard cop who had called me, it was Ophélie. My young friend from the Saint Antoine Institute had sent me a photograph of a guy which seemed to have been cut out of a fashion magazine, with a steely-blue gaze, a shaved head, an unbuttoned white shirt and a predatory smile.

Live from César's, said a brief comment under the picture.

20 out of 20?

That made me smile. I blindly typed in my reply without even slowing down:

Too handsome. Don't trust appearances.

Less than a minute later, Ophélie replied.

Idiot!
And how are you getting on with your pretty redhead?

My heart did a somersault.

My pretty redhead.

Mona.

The image of her warm body against mine invaded my mind without warning.

Her body was probably already wrapped up in a plastic sheet on the back seat of a police car heading for the morgue. I resisted the desire to throw the phone out of the window, to shout into the silence of the night, to put my foot down harder on the accelerator and drive straight at the first plane tree. In the end I merely wedged the mobile under my thigh and concentrated on the road. I was approaching Caen, and I had to avoid the ring road.

The Fiat 500 drove into the village of Grandcamp-Maisy just before three in the morning.

For several kilometres I'd been passing signs announcing 'Omaha

Beach – Liberty Road', inviting drivers to take a pilgrimage between bunkers, shell holes, cemeteries and D-Day museums.

Liberty Road: a funny name for a hopeless journey.

I parked in the church car park and unfolded a road map of Normandy. Isigny-sur-Mer was three kilometres from Grandcamp-Maisy beach, but I was heading for Grandes Carrières, the hamlet where, according to police reports, the body of Myrtille Camus had been found on 26 August 2004.

My finger found the place. I drank another cup of coffee, lukewarm this time, while gazing up at the church, the only illuminated building in the village.

It had been demolished in June 1944, then rebuilt in a hurry. It was a strange building: a concrete cube flanked by a grey, chimney-like bell tower pierced with arrow slits. Even in La Courneuve, the churches had more style than this!

Even in La Courneuve . . .

It was as if someone had projected a hologram inside my mind.

I had seen this church before!

While I'd been driving, scraps of memory had come back to me, the name of the village, Grandcamp-Maisy, this landscape of hedges and stone houses, these slate roofs, this celebration of the June 1944 landings at every crossroads, but my memory had managed to keep them in a bubble of opaque glass.

A bubble that this bell tower had abruptly burst.

I had seen this church before. Once. A long time ago.

And now every detail came back to me.

It was summer. As I did every year, I was supervising at a camp in Clécy, in the Suisse Normande, near Falaise, more than a hundred kilometres from Grandcamp-Maisy. Climbing, canoeing, hiking . . . The kids who attended the leisure centre of the Urban Community of Plaine Commune came from La Courneuve, Aubervillers or Villetaneuse; there were over five hundred them, distributed between camps scattered all over in France. Two of those camps were in Normandy: the one in Clécy that I was helping out at, and another one by the sea, here, in Grandcamp-Maisy. The sea wasn't really my thing, but one of the activity organisers from the sailing camp had needed a day off. Grandmother's funeral or something like that. They were having a lot of trouble finding someone to replace him, and since I had a bit of experience, I was asked to take over. I did the return journey in a single day. Nothing special happened in Grandcamp-Maisy. A swim in that horrible icy water, a bit of teenage flirting on the beach, the occasional reprimand when some of the kids got a bit too big for their boots. That last-minute substitution had vanished from my memory for years. Without that concrete church it would never have come back.

I closed my eyes. Finding the exact date of my last visit seemed impossible. The weather was nice, because we'd had a swim. That meant it was the end of the summer. It was at least ten years ago.

My fingers clenched on the road map.

End of August 2004?

Thursday, 26 August, to be precise?

The day Myrtille Camus was murdered?

Impossible!

The cops had sealed off the area where the body had been found, journalists had hurried to the area. If I had been in Grandcamp at the end of August 2004, a few kilometres from the place where a girl had been found raped and murdered, the teenagers would have talked of nothing else, I'd definitely have remembered.

I opened my eyes and studied the buildings of the hamlet of Grandes Carrières on the map. Four tiny black rectangles.

Except that the Camus case hadn't been made public until the day after the murder. The police had imposed a twenty-four-hour embargo before alerting the media. I hadn't slept on-site, I had gone back to the Suisse Normande late that afternoon. The rape case could have exploded a few years after I passed through Grandcamp, I wouldn't have cared, I wouldn't even have heard of it, I was in Clécy and we lived almost cut off from the world, without newspapers or television . . .

The concrete church lit up in the night taunted me, as terrifying as the watchtower of a concentration camp.

Was it possible?

My trembling hands tried unsuccessfully to fold the road map.

Was it possible that I bumped into Myrtille Camus that day? On the Isigny road, near Grandes Carrières? I was probably driving the Plaine Commune camp minivan, an old Renault Trafic.

I crumpled the map and threw it on the passenger seat.

Was it possible that I had stopped, that I raped her, then strangled her, before my memory erased every trace?

I drank some more coffee, this time straight from the neck of the thermos, and started the engine.

After Osmanville, I turned off along the road leading to the Carrières farm. I passed a large building with beams, mud bricks and closed blue shutters, then continued to the end of the unpaved road.

A new certainty: *I had never been here before.*

The headlights of the Fiat 500 lit up the surroundings. I took the time to study the slightest detail that might jog my memory. Some clue to confirm this madness.

I had come here ten years before, I had abandoned the body of a twenty-year-old girl after murdering her.

Where, exactly?

At the bottom of this little white quarry dug into the limestone? In the cluster of hazelnut trees? To the west, at the foot of that tiny chapel surrounded by the roots of an ancient yew? A few metres further, in one of these fields surrounded by hedges? Or along the Canal de la Vire, which ran for two kilometres from Isigny to the sea?

In the pale halo of the headlights, the sleepy countryside looked like a Millet landscape, but without the angelus, without the prayers, without the farmers who had risen at dawn. Without witnesses, apart from a dozen black-and-white cows that were probably already there browsing the same grass ten years earlier. Mute and indifferent witnesses.

I parked beneath the only streetlamp in the hamlet, about fifty metres before the farm, and got out of the Fiat. I almost expected one of the cows to turn towards me, to recognise me and give me an accusing look.

I was going mad.

I didn't remember anything.

I carried on walking. It was cold, there was hardly any wind. At first I didn't understand why I was heading to the right, towards the undergrowth. For a moment I thought that some phantom memory was guiding me, that my hands and feet were going to reproduce the gestures that my conscious mind refused to admit.

Then I noticed the light. Two lights, to be precise.

Two torches shone at the foot of a hazel tree.

Then I saw the carpet of petals below the torches.

Then I saw the shadow of two panels nailed to the tree.

I couldn't decipher a word from that distance, so I walked closer.

The two flames burned in two little porcelain cups, probably filled with some sort of oil into which wicks had been placed. Apple blossoms in every shade of pink drew the shape of two reclining bodies.

I looked up towards the tree trunk, knowing already what I would read on the two wooden boards.

Morgane Avril 1983–2004
Myrtille Camus 1983–2004

I stood there without moving, without even trying to understand who could have organised this funereal display, or how long the flames had been burning, or how those apple blossoms could have flowered in the middle of winter.

Let alone what it meant.

I just stood there without moving.

I felt a great weariness, as if my arms, my thighs, my leg had lost all their strength. I repressed the desire to lie down on the flowers and sleep, to end it all like that.

Everything was clear.

Morgane Avril 1983–2004
Myrtille Camus 1983–2004

I had killed those two girls. Cornered by the cops, my mind had exploded. I had gone delirious to protect myself. I had invented a suicide, witnesses, endless flight. I had involved Mona in my madness and she had paid with her life, a few hours ago. Other innocents would die if I continued to deny the obvious.

The two names danced in the light of the flames.

Morgane Avril 1983–2004
Myrtille Camus 1983–2004

I couldn't take my feverish eyes off them. My legs were as unsteady as if I was perched on two glass matchsticks. I was going to wait here for the cops to come and get me. My brain was numb. I had barely slept for three days, but it wasn't just fatigue that was dragging me into a kind of white cotton-wool hole. It was a dyke breaking, the last one. The surge of spilled blood could flood my consciousness, I was ready.

I took the King Cobra out of my pocket. I held it against my temple for several long seconds.

My fingers clenched on the icy butt of the revolver, as tight as they would go.

I threw the gun on the bed of apple blossom.

I would wait for my judgement.

Other people would tell me what a monster I was.

I barely heard the shadows approaching behind me, just a few footsteps that stopped ten metres away. One of the shadows spoke in a very low voice, like someone whispering in a church. I knew the voice, I had heard it before, just a few hours before, but my slow-motion mind couldn't recognise it.

'They were only twenty years old. They were so beautiful.'

A woman's voice. I turned around. Carmen Avril was standing behind me. She was wearing trousers and a black jacket, the only colour a thin red thread attached to her buttonhole. She held a sprig of apple blossom between her fingers. Slowly she threw it on one of the beds of petals, the one on the right.

'Morgane had her whole life ahead of her. If only she hadn't bumped into you that night . . . If only . . .'

She fell silent, unable to utter another word. On my left the grass was crushed by lighter footsteps. A slender shadow came forward beneath a hazel tree. It too was dressed in black: a waist-length leather jacket and a charcoal-grey velvet dress. And a thin red thread sewn over her heart.

Océane.

Tears were running down her cheeks.

'You should have murdered me as well that night,' the girl murmured. 'Morgane and I were as one. Two sisters. One heart.'

She too set down near the flames the sprig of apple blossom that she was holding in her hand.

'Yes, Jamal Salaoui, you should have murdered me. Even the worst hunters finish off their prey. A wounded animal never forgets.'

Without thinking, like a sleepwalker, I walked towards the undergrowth to lose myself in the night. My legs barely carried me, I had to lean against each trunk, but I stepped forward as a drunk totters from table to table. Behind me, Carmen and Océane Avril hadn't moved. I saw a kind of brightness towards the edge of the forest, in the fields that stretched towards the sea.

I passed the last curtain of trees. A few dozen metres ahead of me, the silhouette of a woman, motionless in the meadow, was looking at the estuary. She was holding a candelabra. Five fragile flames defying as if by magic the wind that came off the sea.

That silhouette was familiar to me . . .

The blood suddenly stopped circulating in my veins.

'Myrtille was my best friend,' the voice said gently.

The words flew away above the hedges, towards the horizon. A few cries of gulls stabbed the silence.

'Myrtille was an angel. Why take the life of an angel, Jamal?'

She turned around, slowly. I already knew the face of that girl whose gleaming eyes were about to crucify me with grief. Pain without hatred, without a desire for revenge. Just incomprehension in the face of absolute evil.

'Why, Jamal?' she said again.

Then Mona gave me a sad smile which meant that there was no longer anything that she could do for me.

I fell down, right there, knees and palms in the mud. I stayed there for several seconds waiting for the red clay to swallow me, or for one of these women to come and finish me off.

Océane. Carmen.

Mona's ghost

The chapel bell rang, a gloomy chime that lasted a few seconds. Instinctively, I got back up, bent-backed and dirty, as if the clay had dried enough to stiffen each of my limbs. I walked towards the shadow of the chapel with the schist walls, fifty metres to my left.

Curiously, in spite of the sequence of inexplicable events, I knew I wasn't dreaming. My mind had abandoned the hope that I might wake up sweating in the bed of room number 7 in the Sirène, or that I'd fallen asleep at the wheel of the Fiat 500.

The door of the chapel opened abruptly. Neon lights and halogens lit up the interior, so powerful that they dazzled my eyes. I stepped forward, shielding my eyes with both hands. In the tiny nave I made out two prie-dieux in front of an altar decorated with faded flowers. As I got closer, I noticed a few pale oak benches, empty, with red books placed on them. Probably bibles or prayer-books.

The bell rang once more. I held out my hands, red with clay.

'We were supposed to marry on the second of October,' a voice rang out in the chapel. 'Everything was ready. Charles deserved to walk his daughter down the aisle. Louise, to hold in her lap the child that I would have had with Myrtille. If only she hadn't bumped into you.'

Two footsteps rang out on the stone floor. The man's wedding suit appeared in the chapel door. My eyes first saw the red thread in his buttonhole, then rose towards his face.

A face that I knew.

The severe face of Christian Le Medef stared at me, then he repeated, clearly for me:

'Madame Myrtille Camus-Saint-Michel. Sounds good, doesn't it?'
As I fled, I heard the words that he spoke, this time for himself.
'If only I had been there to protect her.'

I walked on, towards the farm with the closed shutters I had passed on my way in. I was going to hammer on the door, shout, beg the occupants to let me in, then to bolt the door so as not to let the ghosts in.

There wasn't a single living being in the farmyard, not even a rooster.

A moment later a dog barked. The ridiculous yapping of a lapdog, not the ferocious animal that you would expect to guard a property. Then a light went on somewhere and the ball of fluff appeared like an arrow. It froze a few metres from my clay-covered legs.

'Arnold!' I exclaimed.

The shih-tzu was wearing a beige pullover with red stripes, the one he had worn in Denise's arms on the morning of Magali Verron's suicide.

'Arnold,' I said again.

The little creature refused to recognise his name. He stared at me with a defiant air, showing his fangs at my slightest movement.

I desperately looked for help from the closed shutters of the farm, then I decided to walk forward, holding out my hand, covered with red clay, to the shih-tzu. The dog's muscles tensed, his mouth open, ready to close on my wrist.

'That's enough!' a voice called from the other end of the farmyard.

The dog hesitated, then gave up and ran in the direction of the voice. Two seconds later he jumped into his mistress's arms. Denise Joubain let go of the cane that she held in her right hand to press him against her.

I met the gaze of the shih-tzu's old mistress, then I turned around again. There was only one direction I could take, the path towards the channel, all other exits were blocked by ghosts.

It felt as though every neuron in my brain was stretching to its absolute limit before snapping. Millions of them at the same time. A safety net breaking, falling into the void, taking all moorings with it. My arms, my legs, my fingers, my neck. I felt my blood slowing in my veins, like an engine that coughs and then, inexorably, slows down before stopping once and for all.

I had to keep going for another few seconds.

Get away. Get away. Flee those ghosts.

I had passed the last hedge, almost feeling my way, when the two men in blue uniforms appeared behind me.

'Don't move, Salaoui.'

Piroz . . .

Of course . . . That's all I needed, at this dance of the living dead.

I turned around, struggling to keep my balance.

The headlights of the police van dazzled me like a rabbit blinded by hunters. The police captain, between light and shadow, was pointing his revolver in my direction. His deputy did the same with his usual lack of conviction. I took three steps back, the canal was only a few metres away.

'Stop! Stop, Salaoui. This is the end of the race.'

I held my hands in the air and stepped back another metre.

'We haven't finished our conversation, Salaoui. You remember? I was asking you a question two days ago. Just before you smashed the model of the *Étoile-de-Noël* over my head.'

To my right, in the distance, I saw the lights of Isigny. The dark canal emerged from the harbour and descended to the sea, like a giant sewer, open to the sky.

'One last time, Salaoui. Did you rape and strangle Morgane Avril and Myrtille Camus ten years ago?'

I closed my eyes. In my brain, the dam broke and images flooded in: my hand grabbing a woman's genitals under a dress, her agitated body escaping me, I was tearing her dress, nailing the woman to the ground under the weight of my body, crushing her breasts, tearing off her panties, freeing my cock, my bloody hands tightening a red cashmere scarf around a white neck, hard, for a long time, until the body gave up. I started again. Once, twice. Mona was watching me, in tears.

I took a step back and, when I cried out, three crows flew off

291

from the field, joining the seagulls in the distance.

'Yes, Piroz! You've won. I raped and strangled them. All three . . .'

The decision to dive into the canal was made for me.

III
Sentencing

Rosny-sous-Bois, 3 August 2014

From: Gérard Calmette, Director of the Disaster Victim Identification Unit (DVIU), Criminal Research Institute of the National Gendarmerie, Rosny-sous-Bois

To: Lieutenant Bertrand Donnadieu, National Gendarmerie, Territorial Brigade of the Territory of Étretat, Seine-Maritime

Dear Lieutenant Donnadieu,

Further to my letter of 22 July 2014 concerning the discovery on Yport beach on 12 July 2014 of three human skeletons.

As agreed, we conducted a thorough examination of all the bones, in particular their DNA.

We were able to solve the first mystery quite quickly, namely the cause of their death. It is identical for all three individuals, whom, as I may remind you, we christened, for the purposes of the investigation, Albert, Bernard and Clovis.

All three were poisoned. Their bones contain traces of muscarine, the toxin extracted from amanita mushrooms, at a concentration which leaves no doubt about the criminal intent. For the record, muscarine is a toxin that is very difficult to conceal in food, and which leads to rapid paralysis of the central nervous system, then an inevitable retardation of the cardiac rhythm.

Also for the record, I should remind you that we have also established beyond reasonable doubt that Albert, Bernard and Clovis died

several years apart. More specifically, Albert died in the summer of 2004; Bernard, between autumn 2004 and winter 2005; Clovis in 2014, between February and March. The most likely hypothesis, therefore, is that they were murdered by the same person, employing the same modus operandi, several years apart. But there is insufficient evidence to confirm this beyond doubt; one might equally speculate that Clovis poisoned Albert and Bernard before taking his own life, or even that Albert murdered Bernard, before going on to be murdered by Clovis.

On this point it is impossible to go any further.

On the other hand, and this is the main purpose of this letter, cross-referencing the DNA of Albert, Bernard, Clovis and the National DNA database sheds new light not only on the identity of these three individuals, but also the resolution of an old case, the double murder of Morgane Avril and Myrtille Camus (known as the 'red-scarf killer' case), which the location of the discovery of these three skeletons, namely the beach below the cliff at Yport, inevitably recalls.

To be precise, the cross-referencing between the DNA of Bernard and Clovis and the NDNAD yielded nothing. The identity of these two individuals remains unknown to the police.

Albert's DNA was not a match of any of the identified samples in the database, but his DNA is not unknown to us. In fact, this an understatement; one might say it is one of the best-known of the last decade. Albert's DNA corresponds beyond any possible doubt to that of the sperm found on the corpses of Morgane Avril and Myrtille Camus. Since the date of Albert's death may be estimated as between June and September 2004, and knowing that Myrtille was raped on 26 August 2004, we may conclude with certainty that Albert died between several days and several weeks after the second crime. This explains why, in spite of the thousands of DNA tests carried out on relatives and residents, the rapist has never been identified, but it does not allow us to establish his identity, or to determine the reasons for his death.

I have also forwarded this data on to Judge Paul-Hugo Lagarde, who will assess whether this information calls into question, in full or in part, the official theory concerning the identity of the double murderer, who, as we both know, was formally unmasked on Saturday, 22 February 2014.

I do not know, Lieutenant, whether this information will allow you to shed more light on this matter. Our men continue to work on this enthralling mystery. Perhaps Albert, Bernard and Clovis have not revealed all that they had to tell us, and we are currently moving in the direction of certain complementary tests. We are obviously willing to carry out any research that you consider useful with regard to recent revelations.

Awaiting an outcome which I hope will be favourable to this investigation, please accept our most cordial regards,

Gérard Calmette
Director, DVIU

37

The hope that I wake up?

The light danced in front of my eyes, an artificial light like that of a fluorescent fish in the depths of a dark ocean, a tiny shining point that began to grow until it occupied the whole of my field of vision.

All I could see was a white square.

It must have been one of those school whiteboards that you write on with erasable felt-tip pens or magnetic letters.

I spotted a little red card stuck to the top of the board. I already knew every word on it.

Carmen Avril, mother of Morgane Avril, president
Frédéric Saint-Michel, fiancé of Myrtille Camus, vice president
Océane Avril, sister of Morgane Avril, secretary
Jeanine Dubois, grandmother of Myrtille Camus, deputy secretary
Alina Masson, best friend of Myrtille Camus, treasurer

Like an artist who appears on the stage after parting a black curtain, Carmen Avril suddenly appeared in front of me. She opened her mouth and her voice echoed in my brain as if her thoughts were replacing mine.

'It isn't difficult, Monsieur Salaoui, to make someone lose their footing so much that they are driven mad. To send all certainties toppling into the void. A very small association is enough, five people at the most, as long as they are determined. As long as they are wedded to the same goal, absolutely and unshakeably. *Never forget.*'

She took a step forward. At least that was what I thought as I watched her face assume immeasurable proportions, as when an actor approaches a camera. Her voice also increased in volume, hammering out beneath my skull halting words that seemed to bounce from one temple to the other.

'I have good news, Monsieur Salaoui: you are neither mad nor dead. But I also have some bad news. We, the members of the Fil Rouge Association, accuse you of the double murder of Morgane Avril and Myrtille Camus.'

As abruptly as it had appeared, Carmen Avril's silhouette melted into the darkness, and old Denise Joubain appeared in her place. Only then did I notice some coloured magnetic letters stuck to the whiteboard. Thirteen letters, to be precise.

DENISE JOUBAIN

Denise looked at me, or at least she looked in my direction, because I was unable to move, unable even to say if I was there, in front of her, to know if I even had a body.

Her voice was shrill.

'You see, my boy, I'm not the only one losing my memory.'

DENISE JOUBAIN

Her wrinkled hands slowly slid the magnetic letters around on the board.

Until they formed a different name.

JEANINE DUBOIS

Her voice trembled again.

'You know everything now, my boy. I only hope I too know the truth before I die. The whole truth. My granddaughter's last words, her last breath. At least you can give me that.'

And with that she disappeared, as if a director had cut to the next scene. A moment later the board was still there, but the letters had changed.

Sixteen letters this time.

CHRISTIAN LEMEDEF

The depressed and unemployed man suddenly appeared in front of the board, as if spat out by the night.

A vague smile at the corner of his lips.

They didn't move, and yet I clearly heard the rasping smoker's voice in my skull, as if he too had pirated my brain.

'Between a fifty-year-old man, worn out and alone, and another man of forty, in love with his twenty-year-old lover, a few months away from building a family, his family, there is more than one letter's difference, Salaoui. There is a life. The one you have stolen from me.'

His long fingers moved around the letters of his name.

CHRISTIAN LEMEDEF

And made another.

FRED SAINTMICHEL

'Le Medef,' the broken voice vibrated in my head. 'It took some nerve, don't you think? Calling an unemployed person Le Medef . . . It was so obvious, so tempting, so brazen . . . But you believed, right until the end . . . When it was all there, in front of your eyes!'

He disappeared in turn.

I was pure spirit, slow, calm, as if bound to a cotton-wool dream, condemned to observe this procession in front of the board without the strength to turn my head, raise an arm or a hand. Did I still have them, lost somewhere in the limbo of a violated memory?

300

Same board.
Different letters.

MONA SALINAS

Mona appeared from nowhere, probably a mousehole.

Her eyes lowered. A faint voice, almost a whisper, and yet mingled, as if amplified, with my thoughts.

'Thank you, Jamal. You found my story moving, you told me just now. I'd like to hear yours now, the true story, Jamal. Not a new invention. Not a new escape.'

MONA SALINAS

She took the first and last letters of her first name, and put the two S's in her surname . . .

ALINA MASSON

'We weren't cheating, Jamal. You had all the clues. All the names, all the letters, all the keys. You just had to look. Put them in the right order. But you didn't see anything . . .'

She disappeared.
I'd had enough of ghosts, I thought.

New flash.
The board.
Six letters.

ARNOLD

The shih-tzu was sleeping below the board, on the floor.
An anonymous hand crossed my field of vision.
Changed the order of three letters.

RONALD

The dog opened an eye and then went back to sleep.
    Total darkness.

38

The true story?

When I woke up, it was still dark and my body was pitching around. For a moment I imagined that I'd drowned, that my body was drifting in the black water at the bottom of the ocean but that, by some miracle, my consciousness had remained intact. Then my right hand touched bottom. Warm. Soft. Gentle.

A mattress . . .

I was lying on a bed.

I went on feeling my way around. The bed base seemed to be fixed into a wooden piece of furniture. I tried to get up. Impossible. My left wrist was trapped in a handcuff fastened to a plank in the wall.

Planks all around me.

A coffin?

The planks were moving.

A coffin in the back of a hearse.

I shivered. I was completely naked on the bed. Apart from that dream, that procession of ghosts in front of the whiteboard, my last memory was the sting of icy water in the channel at Isigny by the sea. My rescuers, because they took me out of the water, had been careful to confiscate my prosthesis. As if the handcuffs weren't enough . . .

I changed position and crouched on the bed. My head, near the partition wall at the end, brushed against a thick fabric and slipped underneath it. My fingers settled on a cold glass wall. A window?

303

A curtain? I pulled on the fabric, and the faint light was enough for me to understand.

Water splashed against the glass.

I was locked in a cabin on a boat.

Later, but it was still night because only a half-moon vaguely illuminated the cabin through the porthole, there was a knock at the door.

My visitor didn't wait for me to invite him in. He pressed the switch and closed the door behind him. The fluorescent light on the ceiling dazzled me. In the white halo I recognised Captain Piroz. He was carrying a bottle of Calvados, two little glasses and a sheet of paper rolled up in a cylinder and tied up in a red ribbon.

'Present,' Piroz said in a low voice.

I understood, even though he didn't say anything, that his nocturnal visit was clandestine in nature. He looked at me, naked on the bed, then stared with disgust at my stump.

'What an idea, throwing yourself into the canal! Damn it, we had to dive in too, to get you out of the water. The water in the Vire couldn't have been ten degrees. You'll forgive us for not asking your permission for stripping you, it was either that or you dying of hypothermia . . .'

I rolled up, hiding my penis under my atrophied leg.

'I'd have to say,' Piroz went on. 'Alina overdid it a bit on the Ambien in the thermos of coffee.'

'Alina?'

'Yep . . . You must remember. The pretty little redhead who had no hesitation about getting it on with a crip? Unless you know her better by the name of Mona?'

Mona. Alina. The hosts of Grandes Carrières appeared before my eyes again. Vague. Uncertain. The bells of the chapel mixed with the yapping of the shih-tzu. Probably the Ambien in the coffee. I tried to sweep them away to concentrate on the present moment.

'Where am I?'

'I imagine you've guessed. On a boat. The *Paramé*, a Dutch *kotter* overhauled by some Bretons. It's barely five in the morning, we set off from Isigny as soon as we fished you out.'

He paused, set down the bottle and the glasses on the bedside table in the bunk, then explained, without my having to ask:

'Heading for Saint-Marcouf! You must recently have discovered the existence of this shitty archipelago, the only islands in the Channel from the Cotentin peninsula to the Belgian border. Just to reassure you, it's not a very long journey, barely seven kilometres, but we're travelling slowly so that we don't get there before dawn.'

I looked in vain for a blanket to cover myself up with.

'What are we doing in Saint-Marcouf?' I snapped.

Piroz gently poured the Calvados into each of the two glasses.

'I think it should look like a trial. Interrogation, confession, preliminary hearing, sentencing. But I think they'll speed up the process. Their goal is to sort everything out between tides.'

'Who are they?'

The captain pushed the cork back in with the flat of his palm and looked at me.

'So you haven't worked it out? They showed you a little video montage just now, to dot the i's and the other letters as well, in order, with earphones plugged in your ears and a screen stuck in front of your nose, but you were clearly still in a daze. To explain it as simply as possible, let's just say that you're dealing with some actors who belong to a troupe called the Fil Rouge, does that mean anything to you? Some of them played themselves, others a random character, but they all had the same goal, my lad. To trap you!'

Trap me?

The events of the previous few days passed in front of me. The coincidences, the things that didn't make sense, the contradictory witness statements . . .

'Nice bit of casting, don't you think?' Piroz insisted. 'Carmen and Océane Avril played themselves. Logically, it seemed a good bet that you would try to meet them. Little Alina inherited the most difficult character, that of Mona, a girl who wasn't exactly a shrinking violet and who was passing through Yport. According to the script, she was to seduce you, and even fuck you if necessary . . .

I confess, I was the one who came up with the idea of the patter about silica in the pebbles. The famous professor of molecular chemistry, Martin Denain, had his villa in Vaucottes broken into a year ago. I was involved in the case, we got on, he had taken an interest in the Morgane Avril case at the time. He left me a set of keys so that I could keep an eye on his second home from time to time. That gave us a credible hideout without even having to ask the permission of this respectable scientist, who never sets foot around here in winter.'

Mona had never been a research scientist.

Mona didn't exist . . .

She was just an avatar created from scratch, played by a girl who had meekly learned her part.

Piroz observed my unease with a hint of sadism, then went on:

'The three other roles called for less intimacy. Poor Frédéric Saint-Michel, Myrtille Camus's fiancé, played the first witness, the depressive Christian Le Medef. Myrtille's grandmother, Grandma Ninja, played the second one, old Denise Joubain, with her dog Ronald under her arm, the one she went and collected after the death of Louise and Charles Camus. It was hard to persuade the last actor, Gilbert Avril, Carmen's brother, but someone had to play the part of my deputy. I wouldn't say he performed the role with any great conviction.'

As soon as Piroz had finished listing the credits, I replied without thinking, without trying to run through my head the number of obvious clues that I'd ignored.

'So why all this stupid circus, for Christ's sake?'

The policeman held out a glass of Calvados. I sniffed it suspiciously.

'The Fil Rouge Association has devoted thousands of hours to tracking down the stranger who was present in Yport on Saturday, 5 June 2004 and Isigny-sur-Mer on Thursday, 26 August 2004. Finally, in 2011, after collecting hundreds of witness statements, a single name came out of the hat. Yours, my boy! Jamal Salaoui. You rented a room at the Caïque holiday cottage on the night of 5 June and spent a day in Grandcamp-Maisy, at Plaine Commune sailing club, on 26 August. QED, Jamal. You're the guilty man . . .'

I sighed with relief. A huge weight had just lifted from my conscience.

This whole performance was entirely based on a misunderstanding!

For now, I didn't bother explaining to Piroz that I had never set foot in Yport before this week, that I'd cancelled that reservation at the holiday cottage because the girl I was planning to spend the weekend with had cancelled on me, and I'd made the return journey from Clécy to Grandcamp without passing through Isigny or even hearing of the murder of Myrtille Camus.

'What a crowd of psychos!' I whistled. 'And you, Piroz, agreed to take part in this masquerade?'

The captain drained his Calvados in one and then smiled at me.

'The idea of the set-up came from Carmen Avril, as I'm sure you can imagine. She persuaded all the others. Put yourself in their shoes for a moment. You're the only possible guilty party, but there's no evidence against you apart from the fact that you were there. Not enough to persuade Judge Lagarde to move his arse after all these years – and I did try, believe me. Even worse, we were getting closer to that fateful date of ten years without a new judicial process, which would mean the case being closed once and for all . . .'

Put yourself in their shoes . . .

Piroz was dissociating himself from the others. I had the curious impression that the captain didn't share their conviction. I pressed him.

'You didn't answer my question, Piroz. Since when have the police involved themselves in this kind of madness to trap a suspect?'

He let one last drop of alcohol pass his lips.

'At first, Jamal, it wasn't so bad. It was just a matter of bringing you back to Yport and putting you in the right state to summon up certain memories in your mind. The performance was supposed to last a day, and had two very precise goals, one for each of your visits to the station. For the first, to collect your DNA, your sperm, your blood, your nails and your pubic hair. For the second, the next day, to trap you and make you confess to both crimes. It was all supposed to stop there. Genetic fingerprints and confessions! We hadn't predicted, you young bastard, that you'd smash my model of the *Étoile-de-Noël* in my face and leg it. From that moment, we had to improvise to maintain our advantage by making you think you were losing your mind.'

If he expected me to apologise for that stupid fucking model, he could forget it. I set the glass of Calvados back down on the bedside table.

'You should drink something, son,' Piroz advised. 'You're freezing. You'll catch your death.'

'It's fine, I'll survive! Since you've collected my sperm and everything else, you've had time to compare them with the DNA of the red-scarf killer, haven't you?' I made a point of putting some irony into my voice. 'I imagine you're going to tell me that my sperm is a match for the rapist you've been trying to catch for ten years. If it weren't, you'd be taking a lot of trouble for nothing.'

Piroz gave me an amused look.

'You're right about one thing, at least, son, I've got the results . . .'

He waved beneath my nose a piece of white paper rolled up and tied with a fuchsia ribbon.

'This piece of paper contains the ultimate proof A fifty-fifty chance. Your hall pass, or a one-way ticket out of here . . . But you're going to have to wait a bit before you get my answer.'

I had the same impression as I had had a few moments before. Piroz no longer seemed to believe in my guilt. Or rather, once again, he was playing cat and mouse with me.

He topped up his Calvados.

'First, I'm going to answer your question, the one you asked a little while ago, about why a police officer like me would have agreed to take part in this masquerade, to the point of summoning you to the police station in Fécamp without any of my colleagues being aware of what you were coming to do there? Well, Salaoui, I'm retiring in three months, so I don't give a damn about any possible repercussions or reproaches from my superiors. Then there's the fact that I've been working on this double murder for almost ten years, and I'd have to admit that without Carmen's crazy idea of putting pressure on you until you betrayed yourself, I didn't have a single piece of evidence to make Lagarde agree to reopen the investigation officially, and make you appear as a witness.'

My fist clenched.

'What the fuck! You just had to ask me. Who says I wouldn't have agreed? I didn't rape those girls! I'd have given you a test tube of my blood or my sperm, and it would all have been over without having to go through this nonsense. In addition, I imagine that confessions obtained by such twisted methods would have no value in front of a judge.'

Piroz studied me, as if impressed by my far-sightedness.

'No legal value, you're right, lad. You're perfectly right. In fact, if I agreed to get involved in Carmen Avril's blasted production, it was for a completely different reason, and I'm the only one who knows what it is.' He raised his glass. 'But as with your DNA results, you're going to have to wait a little so that I can explain. Cheers!'

39

Nice piece of casting, don't you think?

He drained his second glass of Calvados. Without thinking, I picked mine up and did the same. The gut-rot set fire to my palate. I wiped the icy drops that ran along my temples and tried to take stock out loud.

'So, Piroz, to cut a long story short, you were keeping me under surveillance. Mona was watching me, and sending me the brown envelopes that revealed, in homeopathic doses, the tiniest details of the Avril–Camus case. Frédéric Saint-Michel and Grandma Ninja played hide-and-seek to make me doubt everything. You create this character Magali Verron, you invent an identity for her on the internet so that her resemblance to Morgane Avril is disturbing, so that I even end up confusing the two women. But—'

My hand suddenly clenched the empty glass. The image of the girl with the swollen face, the red scarf around her neck, on the beach of Yport, blew up in my face.

'But who threw herself into the void three days ago? Who died that morning?'

'No one, Salaoui.'

'Christ's sake, you're not going to try and take me for a fool again. I was there! She fell from the top of the cliff, right in front of my eyes.'

Piroz gently set his glass back down.

'Have you seen *Vertigo*, Salaoui, the Hitchcock film?'

I shook my head.

'*Vertigo* is the story of a private detective who keeps the wife of one of his friends under surveillance. She has suicidal tendencies and, in the end, she commits suicide by throwing herself off the top of a tower. At least, that's what he thinks. In fact, it's a swindle, a trick set up by the husband – she threw down a dummy instead. The detective had been chosen for only one reason: he suffered from vertigo, so he couldn't witness the beautiful girl's death-plunge as it happened . . .'

'What's that got to do with me?'

'Your wooden leg, idiot! Because of that you couldn't get close enough to the edge of the cliff to see Magali Verron's body crashing to the pebbles. Certainly not in the morning, on a carpet of frosty grass. Basically, the whole of Carmen's twisted idea came out of that, an association of ideas, the cliff at Yport and your gammy leg . . .'

'I saw her throwing herself off the cliff. Then, just afterwards, her blood-drenched corpse on the pebbles . . .'

'*Just afterwards* . . . Be more precise, Salaoui. Forty-seven seconds exactly! Long enough to run to the beach via the Rue Jean-Hélie, to go down the steps by the casino and reach the sea wall. We did the calculations dozens of times, you couldn't have done it in less time than that. Once you were at the bottom, two witnesses whose sincerity you had no reason to doubt confirmed that they had seen Magali's body crash on to the beach.

I looked at Piroz, still without understanding. He was sweating. He looked ill at ease. I could see he was thinking of pouring himself a third glass.

'If I'm not a complete idiot, I imagine it was Océane Avril who played the part of Magali Verron. But there's one detail that escapes me, Piroz, one insignificant detail. If it's all as you say, how did Océane end up on the beach? Did she grow wings?'

'Océane is an amazing girl. Incredibly beautiful. Athletic. And most of all she's determined. Determined to avenge her twin sister. As soon as the plan was set up, almost a year ago now, she began training.'

A strange warmth invaded my belly at the list of Océane's

qualities. My dream girl, I thought again for a moment. An angel who could fly.

'Training for what, for fuck's sake?'

'Base jumping. Leaping from a fixed point like a tower block, a church steeple, a cliff. Do they do it on your estate?'

I didn't reply, I was waiting in disbelief.

'If you want to know the whole thing, Salaoui, base jumps are carried out from a height of a minimum of fifty metres. The cliffs at Yport rise almost one hundred and twenty metres above the beach; so you see, even though she wasn't a professional, Océane wasn't taking all that big a risk.'

'I saw her throw herself off the cliff,' I said, 'the red scarf in her hand, the torn dress—'

'That's the advantage of base jumping. The discipline is practised with an extractor, a little round parachute folded up in a bag with a Velcro fastener. It's also known as a tail pocket, because the bag fits to the shape of the back, less than ten centimetres thick. Quite impressive, almost invisible under a jacket or a coat.'

'Or a torn dress,' I added tonelessly.

'You've got it! What you saw as a dress torn by an attacker required many hours of tailoring. The sexy dress had to conceal the harnesses that ran around her waist and passed between her thighs and shoulders, and of course the tail pocket on her back, freed as soon as she jumped and tugged on her ragged dress. Océane is an excellent actress . . . and she had plenty of ways of distracting your attention, didn't she?'

I didn't reply to the policeman. I couldn't believe it. I couldn't admit such an outlandish truth.

Since we had that conversation, since the end of the whole affair, I've checked. I've watched hundreds of base jump videos on YouTube. I spent a whole night, fascinated, following furious lunatics enjoying themselves in all corners of the world by throwing themselves into the void from the most unlikely places – cathedrals, bridges, telephone masts. I also surfed on specialist equipment sites. Piroz wasn't making anything up. You can buy a tail pocket online, and it takes up less room than a handbag worn on your back.

'A fall lasts less than four seconds,' Piroz went on. 'You must have noticed that the base of the cliff is dotted with dozens of cavities in the chalk, caves of various sizes, enough for someone to hide in there. Even fat Carmen! Forty-seven seconds was more than enough for her to put make-up on Océane's face, blood red, then for her to hide with the tail pocket, in the nearest cave.'

I thought of how I had run desperately to the beach. How I had got to the body, just before Christian Le Medef and Denise Joubain. The body lying there.

'Océane was playing at being dead? Christ, how did she manage to keep it up for so long? We waited for more than ten minutes before you arrived with the police van.'

Piroz could resist it no longer. He poured himself a third glass.

'Remember, Salaoui. It was bitterly cold that morning. And yet, what was the first thing Jeanine did, crazy Denise as you know her?'

Denise's reaction came back to me. It was obvious. How could I have been such an idiot?'

Piroz was triumphant.

'She asked for your jacket to cover Océane's face and torso! Most importantly so that she could breathe easily while you were freezing your balls off!'

Piroz moistened his lips with the shot glass, as if to prolong the pleasure.

'There's just one detail that we didn't predict, and that's that you thought of tossing that red scarf, which we had so carefully placed in your path, at Océane. We improvised. Océane jumped with it. Wrapping it around her daughter's neck, to add a little spice to the scene, was Carmen's idea. That must have thrown you, I guess?'

'You're a bunch of bastards.'

Piroz burst out laughing.

'Glad you're taking it so well!'

While he sipped on his drink, without daring to down it in one, I turned my eye to the rolled-up paper.

My DNA, compared to that of the double killer.

The proof of my innocence, proof that all this lunacy led

313

absolutely nowhere. Unless Piroz had faked the test, as he had with everything else.

'You've gone to a lot of trouble for nothing,' I swaggered. 'With all due respect to the hypocrites of the Fil Rouge, with a special mention for that slut Mona, or Alina, whichever you prefer, you've backed the wrong horse. I'm not the killer. Shame . . . Will you pass on the message?'

I held out my hand, as if to indicate to Piroz that I was waiting for the key to open the handcuff that fastened my right wrist to the wall.

'I don't think you've understood, Salaoui. Whether or not you're the rapist, they don't care. They just want a culprit!'

A shiver ran down my body, from the top of my back to my truncated knee.

'Fuck. What fresh madness do they have up their sleeve?'

'Forcing you to confess, first of all. Then they're going to execute you. For ten years Carmen has dreamed of castrating the man who took her beloved daughter from her. For ten years she's been sharpening Océane's grief like a dagger. For ten years Frédéric Saint-Michel has been holding himself back, like a pressure cooker about to explode. For ten years he has dreamed of nothing more than blowing his own Christian principles sky-high by strangling his fiancée's murderer with his own bare hands.'

'Fuck's sake, Piroz. I'm innocent!'

Piroz gently brought his glass towards mine. The bastard wanted to clink glasses! I didn't react. Without turning a hair, he emptied his glass, throwing his head smartly back.

'I know,' he said at last.

An electric shock ran through every cell in my body.

He knows?

He knows what?

That I'm not guilty?

Piroz slowly untied the ribbon around the scrolled paper, then held it out to me.

'A present, Salaoui. I wouldn't have been displeased to discover that you were the rapist. A pathetic one-legged Arab, that would have simplified matters. But I have to acknowledge the evidence: your DNA isn't a match for the red-scarf killer. You aren't the murderer, son.'

I feverishly consulted the sequence of figures grouped in threes, like the ones I had read in the file of Morgane Avril and Magali Verron. Piroz had no reason to lie to me, this time. I gazed at the view beyond the porthole, the pale night over the sea.

'How long have you known?'

'Since about 5 p.m. this afternoon . . .'

'So why this whole circus, if you had proof of my innocence? That ridiculous shoot-out at Les Ifs? That Grand Guignol production at the Grandes Carrières d'Isigny? Why this trip to Saint-Marcouf, for God's sake?'

Piroz took the sheet with the DNA analysis back from me and rolled it up again.

'Gently, Salaoui. Enjoy the moment. The forces of law and order are on your side. They know you're innocent. They're protecting you. You have nothing more to fear.'

I pulled on my handcuffed wrist.

'Free me, for Christ's sake . . .'

'Calm down. To be honest, I wasn't surprised by this result. I would never say that in front of Carmen Avril, she'd tear my eyes out, but I never believed that your presence in both Yport and Isigny identified you beyond doubt as the perpetrator. While I've been working on the case I've had time to come up with another hypothesis. A more personal one . . . And a more complex one too.'

'Go on then, spill, we've got all night.'

'And tomorrow morning, until high tide at least. You'll see. Let's say that when Carmen Avril tried to sell me her crazed idea of catching you, I leapt at the opportunity.'

'Get to the point, Piroz.'

The captain coughed. 'I used you as bait! I joined in with their scheme because—'

Piroz began to cough again. I thought of the contents of the brown envelopes, the most recent advances in the inquiry, about the doubts of Mona-Alina. Myrtille Camus knew her rapist. She and Morgane Avril were victims of a seducer. They arranged to meet him . . .

I raised my voice.

'Because you had discovered the identity of the real culprit?'

Piroz gestured to me to talk more quietly. I carried on speaking at almost the same volume.

'I know him? The police have checked all the genetic fingerprints of the relatives of Morgane Avril and Myrtille Camus. The double rapist can't possibly be one of them!'

I paused, then asked him another question.

'And what has this prisoner's dilemma nonsense got to do with anything?'

Piroz gave me an enigmatic smile.

'You'll know in a few hours, Salaoui. It's all planned. Everything's in place. Trust me. I only need one favour of you: play their game! Over the last few days they've messed with you enough to keep up the act for another few hours, don't you think? Tomorrow morning, don't talk to them about our little conversation. No one else knows. Your innocence must remain a secret for a few more hours. It's our only way of getting the guilty man to give himself away.'

'Don't you think I've had enough of these idiotic strategies of yours?'

He opened the bottle of Calvados again and poured himself a fourth glass.

'To your health, Salaoui. It'll all be over in a few hours. You will be as white as the driven snow. You'll be able to get it on with little Alina to your heart's content.'

He took a glass from the bedside table and held it out to me, but I didn't move a muscle. Piroz shrugged.

'You've scored a bit of a hit there, son. The more time she's spent with you, the less she's believed in your guilt. Let me give you a piece of advice, Salaoui. Apart from me, she's your only ally on this boat.'

Mona?

My only ally?

316

At that moment I felt the deepest contempt for that sly little mouse.

Illusion. Betrayal. Deception.

To think that Ophélie had given her 21 out of 20 and said:

Don't let her go, she's the woman of your life.

The woman of my life?

My only ally?

I didn't yet know how wrong both Ophélie and Piroz were.

When Piroz left the cabin, taking with him his piece of paper, his bottle and his two glasses, tottering a little, I felt an intense heat rising up, enveloping me, asphyxiating me, as if the wooden slats of the cabin were those of a sauna. Weirdly, I thought of the day when I'd smoked my first joint, all on my own, one Saturday evening, on the roof of the inner courtyard of my middle school. That day I'd severed all the moorings, all the ropes holding the bags of ballast that kept me on the ground.

Free!

I felt light! I was innocent. The police had proof.

All that was left for me was to bid farewell to this troupe of idiots who had almost driven me mad.

With the exception of Océane, perhaps . . .

40

Play their game?

The cries of the cormorants and gulls woke me up, as if thousands of seabirds had met up on social media to welcome the arrival of the *Paramé* in Saint-Marcouf. The day seemed barely to have broken. A timid sun aimed its red eye at the middle of the porthole, lined with tears of foam.

The wooden walls began to vibrate. Shouting, men this time. I understood that they were mooring the *Paramé*. The door of my cabin flew open a moment later. I recognised Carmen Avril by her imposing bulk. She was wearing a large purple waxed jacket.

'It's time,' she exclaimed.

She studied my naked body with revulsion, her eye lingering on the stump of my left knee. She was staring at a monster. A sick and perverted creature. I had rarely observed such a mixture of fascination and hatred in the face of my handicap.

The murder of her beloved daughter. Who she thought . . .

I ostentatiously stretched out on the mattress, opening my thighs to reveal my penis.

I was innocent! The cops were on my side, not hers.

'Put that away,' Carmen growled, throwing a balled-up garment on my bed.

With the same movement, she pointed at me with the iron rod that she was holding behind her back. A kind of poker, but longer and thicker, two centimetres in diameter and a metre long.

Instinctively I retreated into the back of the alcove. I was innocent but handcuffed, naked, defenceless in the face of a madwoman who had been chewing over her vengeance for ten years. Carmen Avril brought the iron bar towards me and held it balanced in front of my face.

Time stopped. For ever.

At last she dropped it to the floor. The iron bar vibrated with an endless echo of cymbals.

'You can use that as a crutch.'

Without another word, she set a small key down on the bedside table, probably the one for my handcuffs, and left the cabin.

As soon as I set foot on the deck of the *Paramé*, wearing the neoprene wetsuit Carmen had tossed on my bed, Frédéric Saint-Michel passed me in silence and went down to the hold. I didn't have time to insult them, to shout at them about how humiliating it was for me to have had to climb the stairs on one leg and keep my balance on the boat, helped only by a metal bar. Frédéric Saint-Michel had already come back up, holding the handcuffs, and gestured to me to hold out my wrists.

Saint-Michel . . . That bastard Xanax! He'd taken a beating over the last ten years, this guy Chichin that all the girls loved . . .

I thought again about Piroz's advice.

It's all planned.

Everything's in place.

Play their game.

I let go of the iron bar and held out my arms. Then I hopped over to a storage bench at the foot of the ship's rail to sit down.

Two fettered hands, one leg. Did they seriously think I planned on swimming back to the mainland?

The *Paramé* was moored on the Île du Large, one of the two islands in the archipelago of Saint-Marcouf. This island, 150 metres by 80, was essentially a fortress built in the middle of the sea. It immediately made me think of *Fort Boyard*, the show that fuelled my fears and fantasies as a kid, with its dwarves, tigers, spiders and the breasts of the starlets in their low-cut swimwear.

The central part of the fort of Saint-Marcouf, a kind of coliseum with a lookout post, was protected by battlements that ran all the way around the citadel, then by thick brick walls almost entirely covered with seaweed or moss. At high tide, the sea must have submerged much of the enclosure. Only the sea wall to which the *Paramé* was moored seemed more recent.

Carmen came and stood right in front of me.

'Don't expect to be rescued, Salaoui. Mooring on the Île du Large has been forbidden for years for security reasons. Only the association that maintains the fort has permission to moor its boats there, but the volunteers don't work in the winter . . . any more than sailing boats venture out on to the Channel.'

I didn't reply. On a table set up on the deck there were cups, a thermos of coffee and pastries. Frédéric Saint-Michel turned towards me, holding a coffee and a croissant.

'A cup of coffee?' he asked me in a glum voice that suggested neither sympathy nor antipathy.

He couldn't have had much difficulty portraying his character; his face bore the same depressive mask as Christian Le Medef's.

'No, thanks,' I replied, loud enough for Mona to understand me. How long would it take before I could call her Alina? 'I'm still suffering from the effects of the last one I drank.'

Mona didn't respond.

She was standing near the prow, turned three-quarters towards the other island, the Île de Terre. Her loose red hair was lashing her face, which was crimson with cold, and perhaps even by some tears that had dried around her swollen lids. Beside her, to starboard, Denise Joubain had put a hand on the rail and with the other she was holding her shih-tzu. Arnold was tearing into a pain au chocolat as if attacking a living prey.

Gilbert Avril was above me, behind the glass of the captain's cabin, checking some sort of nautical measuring equipment.

The least convinced of the troupe, I thought. Even for a seven-kilometre voyage, even in calm weather, he was probably going to find all kinds of excuses not to leave the tiller and let the others get on with the dirty work.

Carmen passed in front of me, poured herself a cup of coffee, not least to warm up her fingers, then she walked past Océane and gave her a beaming smile.

The complicity of those who have emerged victorious after making enormous efforts.

The reward. The apotheosis.

Océane held a cigarette between her fingers, which protruded from a pair of mauve mittens. She had pinned back her hair with some grips of the same colour. Her hairstyle emphasised her features, her dark eyes, giving them the elegance of a Hollywood actress. A beautiful woman on the deck of an ocean liner leaving New York to seduce Paris. Unlike the others, she didn't try to avoid my gaze. She stared at me, every now and again letting the sea breeze carry the smoke between us.

A light veil of mystery. I was left-handed and one-legged, but I felt invincible.

Océane was probing me. She was interested in me. She was wondering. The opportunity was almost too good in the end. Had it not been for that gross misunderstanding, mixing me up with someone else, such a beautiful woman would never have deigned to glance at me.

It's all planned, Piroz had said.

Everything's in place.

Play their game.

The old drunk was the only one who wasn't standing on the deck. He was busy guzzling Calvados, waiting to pull his famous counter-hypothesis out of his sleeve.

The low voice of Frédéric Saint-Michel rang out behind me.

'Shall we get it over with?'

Carmen set down her cup of coffee.

'You're right, let's not waste time, the sea has been rising for two hours.'

I didn't grasp the connection.

'Alina,' she commanded. 'Tighten the moorings.'

Mona reacted mechanically, slowly hauling on the orange buoys wedged between the *Paramé* and the sea wall of the Île du Large. Denise kept Arnold out of the way during the manoeuvre.

'Which one?' Carmen asked, studying the brick wall.

'The third one from the top,' Frédéric Saint-Michel replied, looking in the same direction.

The third what?

I couldn't see anything on the wall but viscous seaweed, some of it soaked by the waves, the rest relatively dry – for a few more minutes.

'The least rusty one,' Carmen said, pointing at a brass ring embedded in the wall, more than a metre above the current level of the sea, but fifty centimetres below its maximum level, judging by the permanent dampness of the seaweed. I immediately understood why they had asked me to put on a neoprene wetsuit.

They planned to tie me to that ring! And wait for the sea to rise.

A trickle of acrid sweat slipped between my skin and the wetsuit.

What was their intention? Make me confess to crimes that I hadn't committed? Force confessions from me and then hand me over to the police? Or would they punish my 'crime' by leaving me there to die?

I thought again of Piroz's advice.

It's all planned. Everything's in place.

I prayed that the police captain wasn't mistaken.

That cop who was still sleeping it off.

Océane flicked her cigarette butt into the sea, then gave me another defiant look. Unfathomable . . .

Carmen came towards me.

'You get it this time, don't you, Salaoui? The sea is rising by about a centimetre a minute . . . Which means you have just over an hour to talk to us about your crimes.'

I gulped down my saliva.

Play their game.

OK, Piroz, I have no choice, but shift yourself.

'And then?' I asked.

'At the end of the hearing, the jury will decide. A jury of the people – I'm sure you don't need me to list the members of the jury. It's in your interest to be convincing.'

Play their game.

'You're a bunch of sickos,' I spat.

Carmen ignored the insult and turned to Frédéric. 'Go and get Piroz! We're going to need another man to chuck Salaoui in the sea, because Gilbert refuses to get his hands dirty.'

Gilbert Avril said nothing. He probably couldn't even hear his sister's words over the cries of the gulls gathered on the roof of the wheelhouse.

Frédéric disappeared into the hold. Mona's hands were still gripping the mooring ropes that were being whipped by the waves. Blue with cold. The thin sunlight of dawn had already been swallowed up in an eiderdown of clouds. The temperature outside couldn't have been more than five degrees. The temperature of the water didn't bear thinking about.

Océane lit a second cigarette. Carmen drained a second cup of coffee.

'What's that idiot doing?' she muttered, when Saint-Michel failed to return.

Eventually his footsteps echoed on the stairs. His face was distorted with bewilderment.

'Piroz isn't in his cabin,' he said.

A yawning chasm opened up beneath me. Fate was dashing me against the walls. The cormorants seemed to mock me with their cries.

'Have you looked anywhere else?' Carmen asked. 'In the head? In the shower?'

'Christ, Carmen, the boat's thirty metres long!' shouted Frédéric, venting his irritation. 'He's gone, I tell you!'

Without a word, Carmen, then Océane, then Denise went down and searched every corner of the *Paramé*.

Without success.

The police captain was no longer on the boat.

Had Piroz drunk too much and fallen overboard? Had he

deliberately jumped into the icy water and set off in an inflatable raft to get help? Or had he been silenced because he knew too much, because he hadn't been careful enough?

While Gilbert Avril, at Carmen's insistence, counted the *Paramé*'s life jackets one by one, I thought of Piroz's words:

No one else knows. Your innocence must remain a secret for a few more hours.

No one else knows.

Gilbert Avril cursed and put all the life jackets back in their box. Not one was missing.

Terrified, I looked at the brass ring fixed to the wall.

The sea had already risen by at least ten centimetres.

41

No one else knows?

'We were knee-deep in the Big Muddy and the big fool said to push on.'

I don't know why, but that old song by Graeme Allwright that we used to sing at camp kept repeating in my head.

In reality, the water was halfway up my thigh. I wasn't cold, not yet, protected by the neoprene. The most painful thing was the dragging of the ring on my arms.

I had tried out different positions, using one hand, then the other, then both to ensure that one shoulder wasn't carrying all my weight. I knew that as soon as the water rose, as soon as my body was floating, I would suffer less.

And before long I wouldn't suffer at all.

Gilbert Avril had helped Carmen and Saint-Michel get me out of the boat and secure my handcuffs to the brass ring in the fortress wall. After cadging a cigarette from Océane, only to throw it away almost immediately, he had grudgingly lent a hand while muttering 'Bullshit' through gritted teeth. As soon as I was chained to my stake, he had gone back to the deck of the *Paramé*.

I didn't struggle. I dismissed the thought of resisting, making their task more difficult by thrashing on the deck like a worm cut in half. What would be the point? It would only add to the humiliation I had already endured.

Besides, there was no escape.

There were six of them. Both Frédéric Saint-Michel and Océane

Avril carried a revolver in their pocket, and they'd made sure I knew it. So here I was, alone. In chains. They hadn't needed to threaten me with their guns, all they had to do was topple me into the cold water, handcuffed, before I was begging to be given some kind of support to hold on to, something that would keep me from going under.

With the precision of a Swiss watch, the water climbed a centimetre a minute. The sea was calm, but that didn't stop the waves crashing against the ramparts of the fort of Saint-Marcouf. The seawater, spraying in my face, made my eyes and mouth salty, and it was impossible for me to wipe it away and ease the irritation. My body lifted with each new wave, before being thrown back against the seaweed-covered wall. I was nothing but a truncated version of a man hanging in the storm being tossed about to the point of exhaustion.

Denise was standing with Arnold on the deck of the *Paramé*, still leaning against the railing. My other torturers had hoisted themselves on to the fortress, sitting or standing on the recently renovated ramparts five metres to my left. From my position I could see only that wall, the top of the central part of the citadel and the watchtower standing out against the cotton-wool sky.

My last hope . . .

The idea had come to me while they were tying me to the brass ring. Perhaps Piroz hadn't been trying to get back to the coast but was hiding on the Île du Large. He was waiting for his moment to appear, perhaps accompanied by a squad of policemen posted in the citadel.

Of the four lunatics of Fil Rouge, Mona – I'd given up trying to think of her as Alina – was the furthest from me, sitting at the end of the rampart.

Deliberately?

Her legs bumped nervously against the wall, as if time seemed interminable. Her wild hair was blown back and forth like windscreen wipers in front of her tear-filled eyes. Saint-Michel was crouched beside her, but he kept getting up every thirty seconds.

He too was nervous. Carmen, rigid and stoic as ever, towered over the others. She hadn't sat down once. She looked away, and then back at her watch.

'Less than an hour, Salaoui. If you want the jury to have time to deliberate before you take your final breath, I advise you to speak.'

The foam exploded in my face.

Only Océane seemed calm. She was sitting cross-legged, her K-Way jacket half covering her jeans. She was still smoking and staring at me without animosity or pity. Just the curiosity of a child watching one insect devour another without trying to save it, because the world is cruel and there is nothing to be done about it.

Incredibly beautiful.

'Speak about what?' I shouted between two waves.

Silence from the jury. I was supposed to confess, without anyone whispering the answers to me.

Fuck's sake, what was that idiot Piroz up to?

The water had risen by another thirty centimetres. It was gripping my chest like a vice.

It's all planned, everything's in place, the police captain's voice hammered in my skull.

Still no sign of him.

'You've got less than half an hour left,' Carmen answered.

Time was moving too fast. A water clock that someone had tampered with. *Fort Boyard*, the snuff movie version.

I spat out a mixture of water and drool.

'OK, I'll tell you everything!'

So much for Piroz, I thought. I couldn't wait any longer. That fat drunk should have let me know when the cavalry was due to arrive.

I yelled to make myself heard above the crashing of the waves.

'You've had it all wrong from the start. I didn't murder Morgane and Myrtille! Piroz knows it – he told me so last night.'

Then I gave them the details, finishing with the DNA results Piroz had been holding in his hand. That piece of paper might still be in his cabin, even now, so would they please get a move on and find it!

'Go and see,' Carmen said to Océane and Saint-Michel.

They got to their feet without a word of dissent.

Meanwhile I went on arguing. Yport, where I had never set foot, in spite of that cottage reservation. That part of Normandy where I had spent one afternoon, long enough to see the concrete church of Grandcamp-Maisy and little else.

Mona didn't even turn her head. She already knew that version. A wave higher than the others lashed my face, drowning my last arguments in a mouthful of salt water that left me retching and helpless.

I was going to die.

I said nothing more. I'd decided not to tell them what Piroz had been up to, his plan to use me as bait to unmask the guilty man.

Could the murderer be someone on this boat?

'I was waist deep,' Graeme Allwright sang.

Océane and Frédéric Saint-Michel reappeared from the hold ten minutes later, empty-handed, shaking their heads.

Nothing. They had looked everywhere.

The copy of the DNA results was nowhere to be found. Piroz had disappeared without taking any steps to protect the one piece of evidence that would prove my innocence. Incompetent fool!

My eyes were being eaten away, stung by thousands of salt crystals.

'Wait, for Christ's sake!' I shouted, my throat spilling over with bile and foam. 'Piroz showed me the sheet of paper last night. It was the regional police records office in Rouen that carried out the analysis. Call them, damn it! They'll confirm the results.'

Océane lit another cigarette and sat down, still indifferent. Saint-Michel took a few steps towards the fortress.

'Don't try and play for time, Salaoui,' Carmen replied. 'You haven't got much left.'

Perhaps twenty minutes . . .

Maximum.

The water came up to my shoulder blades. My position was unbearable. By tensing every muscle to maintain a precarious balance,

I could just about keep my head above water. I could even, with the help of my amputated leg, anticipate the most aggressive waves. The torture devised by Carmen and her friends was remarkably effective. Every effort that I made to cling to life brought me closer to death.

The horizon remained empty.

A few clouds broke. A fine drizzle began to fall on Saint-Macrouf.

With my mouth gaping and eyes wide, I lapped the sweet rainwater that trickled down my face. On the deck of the *Paramé*, Denise and Uncle Gilbert took shelter in the wheelhouse and then disappeared with Arnold into the misted glass cage.

Carmen merely raised the hood of her purple anorak. Saint-Michel opened a black umbrella that didn't look as if it was going to survive the wind for long, and moved over to Mona to offer her shelter. She showed neither gratitude nor irritation.

Only Océane braved the shower.

The rain swept over her face, making her eyeliner and her mauve eyeshadow drip down her cheeks and her mouth, making her look even more beautiful, an oriental icon left out in the rain, its gold and purple fading to compose a marvel painted by the gods.

I couldn't take my eyes off her. Stupidly, I was falling in love. Even though I was going to die in a few minutes, I felt an irrepressible desire for this girl, while she in turn probably desired nothing more than my death. There was some sort of transference at work here, which the shrinks at the Institute would have loved to analyse. I was rapidly losing my mind.

I pulled on the ring to hoist my body out of the water for a few moments, then shouted over the noise of the waves, the gulls and the rain.

'Piroz had another theory! He wanted to trap the real culprit!'

My body fell back into the icy water.

'It wasn't me,' I said at the top of my lungs. 'Not me!'

One last breath. Then I expelled all the air I had left.

'One of you!'

No reaction. Arnold, whom Denise had let out of the cabin, yapped and ran after a cormorant that had settled on the deck.

'Rubbish, Salaoui,' Carmen remarked. 'You've got a quarter of an hour to confess.'

'I was chest deep,' Graeme sang.

'It's all planned, everything's in place,' Piroz replied.

Bastards!

What plan could Piroz have put into action on this rocky outcrop? Why here, in Saint-Marcouf? Because Myrtille Camus had spent the day there once on a boating trip, shortly before she died? What was the connection between Piroz's plan and the doubts expressed by Alina? Myrtille wearing sexy clothes on her day off, Myrtille meeting up with her rapist, Myrtille recording her secrets in a sky-blue Moleskine notebook that no one had ever seen again.

Myrtille and that signature which had bothered Alina: M2O.

So she too knew that I wasn't the killer.

Alina. Mona. The one who had been given the job of seducing me. She was my only ally – that was what Piroz had said.

Alina, a stranger. Mona, a traitor.

My eyes reluctantly abandoned Océane to stare at the girl I couldn't help but call Mona, sheltering under Saint-Michel's umbrella.

My eyes pleaded with her.

Tell them everything, Mona. Tell them. Quickly.

She listened to me without my having to open my mouth, she understood me without a word being exchanged. She rose to her feet, brushing away Saint-Michel's umbrella.

'That's enough,' she said in a low voice that I struggled to hear.

She spoke to Carmen.

'You can see that he's not going to confess. Guilty or innocent, it's not for us to decide. Let's get him out of there and hand him over to the police.'

'They'll let him go,' Carmen snapped. 'Without a confession, they'll let him go.'

Mona wasn't giving up.

'We decided to set ourselves up as a jury. It's the jury that has to decide. We make decisions together, that's what we've always done.

The water cascaded down my shoulders.

Get on with it, for God's sake!

'OK,' Carmen conceded. 'Those who want to take this scum out of the sea, raise your hands.'

Gilbert and Denise, in the cabin, hadn't heard the question, or pretended not to have heard. Océane merely lit a new cigarette without making a gesture of any kind.

Mona looked in turn at each member of Fil Rouge, and then raised her hand.

'For heaven's sake,' she said. 'There's a doubt. We all know there's a doubt. We can't let this boy drown just because we have no one else to avenge ourselves on . . .'

She turned to Saint-Michel. An eternity.

Three more centimetres of water, an icy blade pressing against my Adam's apple.

Saint-Michel did not raise his hand.

'The verdict is in,' Carmen announced. 'One vote to save Salaoui, five against. Sorry, Alina.'

It was over, I'd been condemned.

'I was neck deep,' Graeme Allwright chuckled.

One wave in two smashed against my mouth. I swallowed two out of three. I was coughing. I couldn't breathe.

It's all planned, Piroz had said. *Everything's in place.*

Idiot!

The DNA results had exonerated me, a cop believed I was innocent, but the members of the Fil Rouge couldn't have cared less. They needed to execute someone because one of their own had been executed.

A life for a life.

The cycle of death.

My neck disappeared in the foam.

Suddenly, through the mist, I heard Arnold barking on the

deck of the *Paramé*. Louder and longer than he had barked at the gulls.

Everyone turned round. My eyes opened wide.

Carried by the currents to the Île du Larges, a body bobbed against the hull of the *Paramé*.

Piroz.

He hadn't fallen overboard by chance after one glass too many. He hadn't gone for help either. He was floating on his back like a scarlet raft, with a ridiculous mast sticking out of his heart.

The handle of a knife.

Murdered.

It's all planned, everything's in place, he had told me.

My arse!

We had spoken too loudly in my cabin last night. Piroz hadn't been careful enough. The real culprit had been spying on us. Piroz had been silenced.

By whom?

It didn't matter now. The only thing that mattered was that certainty.

No one else knew.

The only person in the world who had proof of my innocence had been rendered silent for ever. And my death sentence was confirmed.

The members of the Fil Rouge watched Piroz's lifeless corpse drifting into the tiny harbour, bloated with seawater and even stouter than usual.

Everyone except Océane Avril.

Only Océane seemed obsessed by another spot a few metres away, on the brick wall near Mona's foot.

Instinctively I turned my head and tried to work out what it was that she saw.

At first my eyes couldn't decipher it. Then, between two waves, I saw it quite clearly.

You just had to look in the right place.

Océane looked as startled as I was.

Carved on the ochre bricks were two letters and a number, almost erased, initials like those written by lovers to seal their passion for eternity.

M2O

42

One of you?

M2O

I stared in disbelief at the brick.

The two letters and the number stood out in fine white lines carved into the clay, as if Myrtille Camus had come back to Saint-Marcouf to engrave them only a few days before, or someone else had been devotedly coming here for ten years to maintain them.

Spume exploded in my face. I spat out a mixture of cold foam and salt.

In my frantic state, I didn't care how that epitaph had reappeared from the past. The only thing that mattered was its meaning. It was obvious. As violent as a curtain being torn and suddenly revealing the raw truth.

M2O didn't mean 'Marriage 2 October', as everyone had believed.
M2O had a different meaning.
Initials like those written by lovers, I thought again.
Myrtille aime Olivier.
M2O

Myrtille loved Olivier. Olivier Roy, the handsome boy who had prowled around her at the camp in Isigny, off Saint-Marcouf or on the beach at Grandcamp-Maisy, the guy with the white and blue Adidas cap that Commander Bastinet's forces had been looking for. Olivier Roy who had disappeared on 6 October 2004.

Alina had been mistaken when she had given her statement to

the police. Olivier Roy hadn't been hanging around Myrtille Camus because he was a pervert eyeing up his potential prey . . . No! The reason was much simpler: Myrtille and Olivier were sleeping together. They were having a summer romance, and Myrtille, a few months away from her wedding, hadn't dared to say a word to her best friend . . . Alina had suspected for all these years, but she could never bring herself to acknowledge it.

The sea covered my chin. My body trembled with cold and a nervous energy. The adrenaline was speeding up my thoughts. Everything I'd discovered over the last few days passed in front of me. Commander Bastinet and Ellen Nilsson's investigation.

M2O

Myrtille loves Olivier.

Those verses danced in my memory . . .

I will put grilles on the universe
To keep it from parting us

I will dress our good fortune in rags
To keep it from buying us

I will kill all the other girls
To keep them from loving you

M2O

That poem had been written for Olivier Roy, not for Frédéric Saint-Michel . . .

With one desperate movement, I pulled on my arms to lift myself above the water for a moment. I filled my lungs and then I yelled:

'There!'

My cry was accompanied by Océane's pointing finger.

The members of the Fil Rouge froze. Captain Piroz's water-bloated body sank against the sea wall of the fort of Saint-Marcouf and then, like a stubborn balloon, bumped against the wall with each rise and fall of the waves. No one paid it the slightest attention.

Mona scrambled down to the edge of the rampart and reached out her hands to the carved stone, a metre above sea level. The brick wasn't embedded in the wall.

Gently, Mona's right hand slipped the stone from its place, revealing a cavity about ten centimetres deep. She leaned further forward. Her left hand blindly explored the gap in the wall. A second later, she took out a transparent plastic bag.

The water was licking my lower lip. In another minute it would engulf my mouth. As a new wave submerged my face, I glimpsed a sky-blue rectangle under the cellophane.

Was this Piroz's surprise?

Everything's in place, he had said.

Had he staged this moment? Carved the stone and hidden the bag?

Mona tore open the plastic with her teeth. The transparent scraps floated away in the wind while her fingers clutched the little blue book.

A Moleskine notebook. Myrtille's notebook, the one in which she had recorded her most intimate feelings.

Later, when I replayed every detail of that scene, I would list the sum total of coincidences, the reaction of each member of the Fil Rouge, their precise location on the deck of the *Paramé* or on the rampart of the Île du Large, and I would arrive at a logical explanation. The inevitable outcome of a long, very long wait. But at the time my brain was screaming out a single order:

Mona, get a move on!

The water was gnawing at my nostrils. Lactic acid burned my shoulder muscles. But I tensed my deltoids to hoist myself above the waterline, keeping my chin above the water. When the pain became too intense, I breathed in, relaxed, held my breath and plunged my head under the sea for several seconds, releasing my muscles before tensing them again to emerge into the air. How long could I keep this going?

Mona was reading the notebook. Only her lips moved. In perspective, her silhouette stood out against the white sky, topped by the watchtower of the fortress.

'So, Alina?' Denise's voice rang out from the deck of the boat.

Arnold barked.

Frédéric Saint-Michel thrust his hand into the pocket of his jacket.

Carmen and Océane were standing side by side, their matching K-Way waterproofs forming a single mauve plastic sheet. Mother and daughter didn't seem to have grasped the sequence of events.

I went under again. Counted to thirty.

My head broke free of the water.

Mona looked up from the notebook and stared at Frédéric Saint-Michel. Her voice seemed far away, almost unreal, filtered by litres of seawater.

'She wanted to leave you, Frédéric. Myrtille didn't love you any more—'

'Nonsense!' Saint-Michel shouted.

Carmen stepped forward, but Océane held her back. Mona looked down at the Moleskine again. It took her an eternity to turn the page.

Mona, please!

The sea swallowed me up again. This time I stayed down for twenty seconds. Then, braced against the brass ring, I appeared again, gasping for oxygen until my lungs felt as if they would burst.

Mona's voice dragged, further and further away.

'She had met someone else, Frédéric. Someone who had opened her eyes. Who had given her the courage to face her family. Charles and Louise. Me. Courage to refuse what everyone expected of her—'

'Bullshit!' yelled Saint-Michel's.

Piroz's corpse had drifted and was now floating two metres away from me. I looked at it, my strength waning. The wave struck me full in the face, open-mouthed. I thought the ocean was filling me up. I was drowning, unable to spit out a word, and no one was paying me the slightest attention.

Everyone was waiting for Mona to speak.

'They're her last words, Frédéric. The last words she wrote in this notebook.'

The words swirled. My leg, the only muscle still capable of resistance, pressed desperately against the wall, my toenails under the water seeking a gap between two bricks.

Support yourself. Gain a few seconds at the cost of an unstable balance that the smallest wave might overturn.

My foot beat around in the void without finding the slightest purchase.

I couldn't get my head out of the water.

I closed my eyelids and my mouth, holding my breath for ever. A few centimetres from the surface, as if in a bubble, I heard Mona's voice:

'"August twenty-fifth. Three o'clock in the morning. Fred arrives tomorrow. It's my day off. I insisted on him coming. He can't admit that it's all over. I arranged to meet him in a secluded spot, beside the Grandes Carrières farm near Isigny. I hope he'll understand this time. I hope Mum, Dad and Alina will understand. I hope I won't disappoint them all. I hope it will be over with quickly. I can't wait, I really can't wait, to see you again, Olivier."'

I opened my eyes. My thoracic cage was about to implode. I could see only vague shadows across the water.

Mona stepped towards Saint-Michel.

'You were in Isigny, Frédéric? At the Grandes Carrières? The day Myrtille was killed?'

The shapeless outline of Saint-Michel leaned forward, extending his arm and pointing it in my direction.

'This is all a trick, for God's sake. He's the killer. Him!'

I worked out too late that Saint-Michel was holding a gun in his hand, that he was about to fire it at me.

I dipped back under the water, but my wrists, cuffed to the ring, held me less than fifty centimetres below the surface.

An ideal target . . .

Then everything happened very quickly.

'Die!' Saint-Michel yelled.

Then I heard Océane shouting: 'No!' Followed by the shot.

I waited for the bullet to pierce my body.

Nothing.

Three more shots rang out and then, a moment later, Frédéric Saint-Michel's body toppled from the rampart, five metres away from me, while Océane screamed.

I worked out that she had been faster on the draw, that she had shot first. Then a second time and a third, at the murderer of Myrtille Camus. The murderer of her sister Morgane.

A second later, the surface was disturbed once more.

Mona had dived in.

I felt her body pressing against mine, her mouth settling on mine and kissing me to grant me a reprieve several seconds long, a few extra breaths. She rose from the water, took a deep breath, plunged below the surface and kissed me once more while her feverish fingers clung to the brass ring.

I heard the metal click of rattling keys, then the handcuffs opened.

I was free! Alive. Innocent.

From the deck of the *Paramé*, Uncle Gilbert, his face expressionless, threw us two orange lifebelts.

On the island, Océane was weeping in the arms of Carmen, who sat straight as a rock on the rampart, her great bulk concealing half of the fort.

Mona, drenched in her Kaporal jeans and her green jumper, pressed against me and tried to kiss me again. She only touched a corner of my temple, a mixture of hair and seaweed.

I had turned away. I was just a piece of cold wood drifting away from the lies.

Mona had betrayed me.

She wasn't the one who had saved me.

Clinging to the rope ladder hanging from the side of the *Paramé*, I turned my eyes towards Océane again.

She had raised her head, and was holding my gaze.

Her eyes were the same as they had been a few days before, at the top of the cliff, before she threw herself into the void.

The eyes of the abyss.

A revolver lay at her feet, on the rampart.

Océane had just killed a man so that I could live.

43

A trick, for God's sake?

The beach at Grandcamp-Maisy was still a good kilometre away, but I could already make out the pale façades of the houses on the seafront, lined up like the white teeth of a huge, broad smile.

Carmen Avril had phoned the police. They were waiting for us in the harbour. They would be there before us, they had assured us, even though the crossing from Saint-Marcouf took only a few minutes. They would probably mobilise all the brigades of the area to welcome us. Behind us, the Île du Large had already disappeared in the morning mist. Only the flight of the cormorants above the empty sea suggested that there was land a few wingbeats away.

I was sitting on the storage seat. No one had thought to give me back my prosthesis. Océane was sobbing, pressed against me. Carmen, on the telephone, had entrusted her daughter to me without giving me a choice. I was drenched. The water had finally slipped between the neoprene wetsuit and my skin to settle there, icy and further chilled by the landward wind that stung our faces.

I wouldn't have swapped places for the world.

I wouldn't have made the slightest movement to shelter from the breeze, to wipe away the icy streams trickling down my torso, my arms and my legs, the slightest movement that might have altered this miraculous balance.

Océane's face resting on my shoulder. Her hand around my waist. Her hot tears on my neck, a few burning droplets in an icy torrent.

Prostrate.

Océane hadn't seen Gilbert and Carmen Avril, after many minutes of effort, hoisting the corpses of Piroz and Saint-Michel on to the deck of the *Paramé*. Or Gilbert carting them down to the hold all by himself, with a Marlboro wedged between his lips.

'I knew this was a stupid idea,' was all he had managed to mutter to his sister. Then he had gone back to the wheelhouse and fired up the engine.

Carmen ignored him; she had her ear and mouth pressed to her mobile phone, probably the cops. The crossing wouldn't be long enough to explain to them why the Dutch *kotter* was bringing back two corpses in the hold.

A cop and a murderer.

Mona was sitting against the railing, near the prow. She was staring at the white sky towards the steeple of the church at Grandcamp, the only elevated point on the coast to which a prayer could be directed. Her eyes were red. Denise had tied Arnold's lead to her leg, and was running her hand through his fur. Mona would need some time. Her best friend had been murdered by a man she had known since childhood. Chichin. The man her parents, Charles and Louise, had entrusted with their daughter's happiness.

All gone, buried beneath an avalanche of lies.

All but her.

The waves rocked Océane. I had hardly ever held a baby in my arms, but I understood fathers who could hold a child to their chest for whole nights. I understood that incredible feeling of responsibility that meant you must do nothing, just wait, frozen like a statue for ever. That being there was enough.

Only my thoughts were free to wander. Before we entered Grandcamp harbour, they lost themselves in the void. I had understood nothing, or hardly anything, but the fact that Frédéric Saint-Michel was the double rapist, the red-scarf killer that the police had been pursuing for ten years, that Piroz had worked it out and set a trap for him.

*

Along the endless concrete sea wall that isolated Grandcamp beach from the village, I watched the three police squad cars driving towards the harbour. Probably hanging on Carmen's words.

They'd been waiting for ten years. And now everything was moving very quickly.

They didn't yet know how quickly, and neither did I.

Before the end of the afternoon, the police had carried out the first forensic tests on the Moleskine notebook found behind a brick on the island of Saint-Marcouf and certified beyond doubt that it had been written by Myrtille Camus ten years previously. Other officers combed through Frédéric Saint-Michel's movements on 26 August 2004. A clerk at Elbeuf town hall recalled that the day before the murder of his fiancée, the director of Puchot leisure centre had cancelled meetings with parents to visit possible future sites for adventure camps. Holiday cottages. Sailing schools. Pony clubs. No one had checked, no one had paid any attention at the time.

They were dealing with a serial killer. Who could have imagined that Frédéric Saint-Michel had travelled from Elbeuf to Isigny and back in a day, three hundred and sixty kilometres, to rape his future fiancée?

Before the end of the evening, at about eleven o'clock, the police from the Elbeuf brigade, armed with a warrant from Judge Lagarde, had searched the apartment of Frédéric Saint-Michel on Rue Sainte-Cécile. Hidden away in a locked drawer, they found Morgane Avril's handbag.

It was then that they called the judge to announce that they had finally established the connection between the Avril and Camus cases.

At about midnight, having been contacted by trainee officer Hachani, Sandra Fontaine, a former activity leader at the Puchot centre and now a teacher in Thuit-Simer, above Elbeuf, recalled having talked to her boss about the Riff on the Cliff festival, and in particular about a group that had passed through Yport that evening. Everyone in the region had been talking about the festival that day. Not about the line-up, but about the girl who had been found raped, strangled and thrown from the top of Yport cliff.

At about one o'clock in the morning a group of three officers, led by Commander Weissman of Rouen regional crime squad, settled down to spend the rest of the night writing up their preliminary report.

In all likelihood, Frédéric Saint-Michel had gone to the Riff on the Cliff festival on his own, and had fallen for the charms of Morgane Avril, who had been setting the Sea View dance floor alight. They had left the club together. At some point after that, Saint-Michel had raped the girl, then strangled her. He taken one souvenir home to Elbeuf: the handbag that the police were looking for.

What happened months later, when Myrtille Camus, his fiancée, arranged to meet him at the Grandes Carrières to tell him she wanted to split up with him? Another fit of rage? A Machiavellian plan minutely prepared in advance? Probably they would never know, but Frédéric Saint-Michel followed the same modus operandi as he had for the first murder. Torn dress. Red Burberry scarf used to strangle the victim. That was how he managed to avert the suspicions of the police. The killer was a vagrant, a pervert. Certainly not the fiancé of one of the girls . . .

At three in the morning, Commander Weissman allowed his colleagues a break and tried to wake up Commander Léo Bastinet, who had retired five years ago to somewhere near Ambert, in the Puy-de-Dôme, to inform him about the final twist in the Avril–Camus case. Commander Bastinet picked up after ten rings or so, and hung up before Weissman could get a word in. This was not the case with Ellen Nilsson, whom Weissman managed to contact a few minutes later.

At 6 a.m., the criminal psychologist gave her first televised interview, her hair tousled as if she had just jumped out of bed, her face unwrinkled and free of make-up, her enhanced breasts visible under a see-through silk blouse that she had 'slipped on in a hurry'. She told the journalist, who was staring at her bare legs, that she had always been convinced that Myrtille Camus knew her murderer, but, alas, no one had listened to her.

By ten in the morning, the switchboard operators of Rouen regional crime squad had collected five new witness statements from former activity leaders who'd worked under the supervision of Frédéric Saint-Michel. They all said that when he was in charge of the summer camps, the handsome Chichin had been drawn to the young and pretty trainee youth leaders, and had drawn up an impressive list of groupies, aged between seventeen and twenty, willing to follow him even under the duvet. Several girls admitted succumbing to the guitarist's advances, and described the metamorphosis of the seducer as soon as they had laid down their arms: the attentive romantic in the evening became a ruthless lover at dawn. In a hurry. Indifferent. On the other hand, the police hadn't manged to find a single girl who had passed through Saint-Michel's bed after the summer of 2003, when he was officially going out with Myrtille Camus. Had Saint-Michel found the love of his life? The one he couldn't bear to lose?

Gilbert Avril steered firmly to starboard. The *Paramé* turned towards the harbour, straight towards the concrete jetty that dominated the narrow entrance to the canal. In spite of the early hour, rubberneckers were already gathering on the sea wall. Probably people who lived on the seafront, alerted by the procession of police vans.

They watched us curiously, pointing in our direction, laughing or whispering. Several flashes went off.

Océane, still wrapped in my arms, turned her back on them. The *Paramé* slipped gently over the calm water. I guessed that the storm would break as soon as we pulled in. Two police officers would take charge of each member of the Fil Rouge.

They would be taken to the nearest station and interrogated separately. Packs of journalists were setting up camp in front of the police station.

I took advantage of the last few seconds of calm to list in my head all the doubts that the death of Saint-Michel hadn't laid to rest.

Who had put Myrtille Camus's private diary on the island of Saint-Marcouf? Was it Piroz, in the hope of exposing Frédéric Saint-Michel, as he had implied in the hold of the *Paramé*? But if he had laid his hand on a piece of evidence as crucial as that private diary, why hadn't he directly accused Saint-Michel? If Piroz had guessed the real significance of the signature M2O, why agree to take part in this crazy set-up conceived by Carman Avril, until that macabre dénouement on the island of Saint-Marcouf?

Everything's in place, the captain had said.

What had Piroz planned before Saint-Michel had stabbed him? What did this case have to do with the theory of the prisoner's dilemma to which the captain had attached so much importance?

The Dutch *kotter* skimmed past the end of the jetty. A guy in a sailor's hat was perched on the guardrail, armed with a camera fitted with a telephoto lens. He waved his arms at us. *Jerk!*

Instinctively, I turned to hide Océane's face. The sight of the pack massing on the dock had me panicking.

Océane had killed a man. But Frédéric Saint-Michel was guilty, there was no doubt—

Except there was. The reason Saint-Michel had never come under suspicion until now.

His DNA.

The police had checked the DNA of everyone connected with Myrtille, including Frédéric Saint-Michel. It was not a match for the sperm found on the bodies of Morgane and Myrtille.

Had the handsome Chichin also fallen victim to a conspiracy? Or had he come up with the most ingenious sleight of hand?

None of us knew at the time, but the police would find the solution the following day, at 1 p.m.

A solution as simple as it was obvious . . .

44

Had he found the love of his life?

By midnight, sixty-three sealed plastic bags had been delivered to the regional crime squad in Rouen. Glasses, bottles, knives, forks, toothbrushes, combs, clothes, shoes, glasses, gloves, handkerchiefs, pens, keys, guitar capos, MP3 headphones . . .

The officers from the Elbeuf brigade had obeyed the strict orders of Commander Weissman and painstakingly collected from Frédéric Saint-Michel's apartment all the objects that might contain traces of his DNA.

After sifting through these items, in the early hours of the morning they came upon a glass bottle that contained residues of sperm. A few hours later, a computer spat out a genetic code.

For several minutes the police checked every letter, every number, like players of the lottery who don't dare to believe that they are holding the winning ticket in their hands. They'd been waiting for the right combination for ten years . . .

Then they exploded with joy.

The sperm in the bottle was the same as that found on the bodies of Morgane Avril and Myrtille Camus!

In his report for Judge Lagarde, Weissman hypothesised that Frédéric Saint-Michel had got hold of a stranger's sperm to avert suspicion. That certainty resolved the case while making it even more sordid. Chichin was no longer a lover who had panicked in the face of the about-turns of his two girlfriends, he had been unmasked as a sadistic killer who had minutely planned his o murders. While a police medical examiner, Dr Courade, stated that it struck him as impossible for the sperm found in Morgane Avril's vagina to have been introduced artificially, no one dwelled on that detail. Frédéric Saint-Michel, even with three bullets in his belly, entered the pantheon of Machiavellian murderers.

The *Paramé* entered the harbour of Grandcamp-Maisy. It passed by a dozen colourful trawlers floating idly in front of the quay. The cops thronging the quay looked as though they'd been dumped from the net of some fishing boat in readiness for the auction.

Denise threw a rope to the nearest policeman. The *Paramé* crushed the yellow buoys as it came to rest against the brick quay.

'They want to talk to you,' Carmen said into Océane's ear. 'They want to talk to all of us. But you first.'

A worried voice. Telephone clutched in her fist.

Océane's moist eyes looked away from her mother's and back to me. A band of rain moving in, warm this time. Of course she would have to explain herself to the police. She had killed a man. Three bullets to the body, less than thirty minutes before.

To take her revenge.

To save me . . .

Her hand slipped slowly around my arm.

'I'm sorry, Jamal,' she said. 'Forgive us, it was—'

'They're waiting for you,' Carmen cut in before she could finish.

Océane got to her feet. I thought I saw an expression of regret in her eyes.

'They're calling us,' she murmured.

They're calling us.

While Carmen and Océane disappeared into the back of the blue Renault Trafic parked opposite the *Paramé*, other officers climbed aboard the *kotter*. Some wore latex gloves and transparent plastic hoods. I was still sitting on the chained storage bench and no one seemed to be interested in me. Right in my field of vision, still leaning against the railing, Mona said a quick word to the policeman who was coming towards her.

Too far. Impossible to hear.

The officer nodded and walked away. A second later, Mona came and stood in front of me.

'Hello, Jamal. Since I died near the station at Les Ifs, we haven't had had much of a chance to talk.'

Her laughter sounded false. Hollow, in fact. I looked back at her, stony-faced.

She pursed her lips. The wind was tugging at her red hair, pulling it free of the hood.

'I'm sorry, Jamal. You had nothing to do with any of this. We were all set up. All of us.'

Cold water was still trickling under my wetsuit. I wanted to get it all over with. To give my statement to the police, sign it and get out of there.

'You won't care,' Mona went on, 'if I tell you I didn't agree with them. But I didn't have any choice.'

I turned my head. Carmen had got out of the Renault Trafic accompanied by a policewoman. Not Océane.

'But you see, in the end Carmen Avril was right. So was Piroz. To bring the truth back to the surface, we had to dig up the past.'

Dig up the past?

Bring the truth back to the surface?

Two corpses were rotting in the hold of the *Paramé* – and probably not the ones they'd planned from the start.

A policeman came towards us, his cap pulled down to his eyebrows. Before he was able to say a word, Denise intercepted him, pressing Arnold into his arms. Mona had clearly enlisted help in buying time to talk to me.

What was she hoping?

A stray tendril brushed her lips, and she pushed it away with a grimace. She no longer reminded me of a frightened mouse.

'Jamal, I worked out very quickly that you were innocent—'

Very quickly?

Explain, my pretty one . . .

After we slept together? Before? Afterwards? During?

I noticed a fourth policeman going down into the hold of the *kotter*.

'I had to carry on playing my role to its conclusion,' Mona pleaded. 'In memory of Myrtille . . . of Louise, of Charles . . . It was, how can I put it, unreal. You remember, last night, in the Fiat, in Vaucottes, when you read about the little girl from Puchot and her childhood friend. Mimy and Lina. The desperately sad life of a girl weeping beside you as you read that letter from a stranger . . .'

Last night. At ten o'clock. I felt as if a whole year had passed in the meantime.

Vaucottes. The Fiat. A brown envelope.

'Moving?' she had asked me. 'Thanks,' she had added.

I hadn't understood.

'I remember. You made a fool of me.'

'No, Jamal—'

'Yes . . . Hats off. You're an incredible actress.'

She twisted a red curl between her fingers, hopped on tiptoe like a shy schoolgirl and then took a deep breath.

'No, Jamal. I was sincere. Contrary to appearances, I was sincere. Absolutely sincere. You won't believe me, Jamal, I'm under no illusions, but I have to say it to you. Now. Apart from the thing about the double murder, never . . .'

She finished her declaration under her breath.

'. . . never have I been so sincere in a relationship.'

Her clumsy smile pressed against my face.

Sincere?

Apart from the thing about the double murder?

Apart from the brown envelopes strewn in my path.

Apart from that nocturnal trip to Le Medef's house. Apart from the visit to the bedroom of those traumatised children in the old railway station. Apart from the invented life of Magali Verron. Apart from the dreamed-up life of one Mona Salinas, pebble-collector, holder of a doctorate in silicon, the favourite student of a thesis director who ran the biggest chemistry lab in France, who gave her the use of his villa. Why sell yourself short, eh, Mona? Since you have no choice, why not act the part of a funny, intelligent and overqualified girl . . . And take every opportunity to seduce the sucker sitting opposite over dinner at the Sirène.

'None of it was true,' I murmured. 'None of it.'

'Neither true nor false, Jamal . . . We both made things up, we told each other stories.'

A muted cry rang out:

'Leave me alone!'

In the wheelhouse of the *Paramé*, Gilbert Avril was shouting at a policeman who was trying to pull him away from the tiller. Crazed gulls flew from one mast to the other.

My eye passed over Mona's shoulders.

'No. I believed it.'

A silence.

I saw Océane getting out of the Renault Trafic, escorted by two policemen, then she disappeared into the back of a van. A few minutes later, the van departed.

I had butterflies in my stomach. I averted my eyes.

'I believed it, Mona,' I said again. 'You notice that? I still call you "Mona". Pathetic, isn't it? Mona Salinas doesn't exist. Never has. You are . . . a stranger!'

'If that's what you think . . .' she said after a long pause. 'But Alina's not so different from Mona. She's the same girl, Jamal. The only difference is the order of the letters. We were all playing our part in the end.'

She stepped forward and kissed me on the cheek. She was trembling. She forced a smile.

'I can't be angry with you. That would be too much, wouldn't it? So no hard feelings . . .'

I didn't react. I had nothing to say to her. Mona's cheerful tone struck me as completely fake.

'You remember our first meeting, Jamal? Our dinner *à deux* at the Sirène. I had asked you if you would give me one of your visiting cards, the ones that you handed out to the prettiest girls in the street?'

'I said yes.'

'That's true. But do you remember what I said?'

No idea.

My eyes drifted to the place where the van carrying Océane's had disappeared behind the cream pavilion by the quay.

'I said: "I'm sure that you wouldn't have given me your card. I reckon you go for romantic women, femmes fatales. Not direct girls like me." Mona ran a cold finger down my cheek. "If you ask me, that's the problem with your technique: you collect women like Panini stickers, but you don't get the ones you need."'

A flash of light made me blink. A policeman was taking photographs of the railing of the *Paramé*, probably to find from which spot on the deck Saint-Michel had thrown Piroz overboard. None of them seemed to be in a hurry to question me.

Mona's words slipped around my head.

You go for romantic women, femmes fatales.

You don't get the ones you need.

I remembered now, she had said that on the first evening. I hadn't paid the slightest attention.

'No hard feelings,' I confirmed in a loud voice. 'You were right, Mona, I'm attracted by the stars.'

My hand moved through the empty space beneath my left knee.

'The ones I must conquer! The inaccessible peaks. To climb Mont Blanc, that sort of nonsense. I'm training hard for that.'

'I know. I've always known. Ciao, Jamal. The police are waiting for us. I think we can both bury Mona once and for all . . .'

Alina. I had to get that name into my head.

She twisted around to remove something from her jeans pocket.

'Talking about those inaccessible peaks, I found this yesterday. I'd put it on the bonnet of the Fiat near the old railway station. It fell off when you made your getaway. You may even have driven over it . . .'

Mona slipped my sheriff's star into my hand. Black with mud. Battered.

'You entrusted it to me. You'll have to find another keeper for it.'

I raised my eyes to the sky. Above the crescent moon that frayed into long white clouds, one last constellation twinkled.

'Thanks, Mona. But I don't need it any more.'

Once again I studied the morning stars, hiding coquettishly behind a thin veil of mist, then I took the sheriff's star between my thumb and index finger.

I resolutely flung it as far as possible into the water.

The scrap of gilded metal flew for a moment in an elegant curve, until it bounced on the black water of the harbour.

'You shouldn't have done that,' Mona protested. 'It was your talisman . . .'

The sheriff's star sank gently.

'Your lucky charm,' she added.

She walked away. By the time she'd climbed down three rungs of the ladder of the *Paramé* to get to the quay, a cop in a leather jacket was taking his hands out of his pockets to help her.

On the deck, four police officers appeared, carrying the corpses of Piroz and Saint-Michel wrapped up in opaque plastic bags.

A policeman turned his head indifferently towards me. Perhaps he was hoping I would help them shift the corpses.

I closed my eyes, letting the waves rock me.

Five verbs danced in my head.

Five commandments.

1. *Become* – the first disabled athlete to run the Mont Blanc Ultra-Trail.
2. *Make* – love to a woman more beautiful than me.
3. *Have* – a child.
4. *Be* – mourned by a woman when I die.
5. *Pay* – my debt before I die.

I hadn't been bluffing, not this time.

I no longer needed a star to guide me. I touched each of my five points with my finger. The first was only a question of training. The second was no longer an inaccessible Everest.

Océane . . .

353

Never had I so desired that the same woman would fulfil three of my vows. As to the fifth, I had brushed with death so often that it would wearily grant me a long respite . . .

I've no idea how long I stayed on the storage seat, lost in my thoughts, before a cop came to question me. He was young and smiling, he looked like a trainee. He held out a blanket, asking if I wanted to change. I nodded.

'Follow me . . .'

I got up and hopped on my one leg. The trainee turned, embarrassed. He looked around him as if hoping he would find my missing half-leg on the *kotter*. I half expected him to peer over the side to see if a crocodile wasn't waiting with gaping jaws to devour my other leg.

Then I sensed his embarrassment turning to unease. He looked back at my face.

Suspiciously.

Perhaps he too had difficulty believing that the little one-legged Arab was completely innocent in this affair. No smoke without fire . . . After all, the Fil Rouge had assembled the evidence. I was the only person who had been in the wrong place at the wrong time on two occasions, putting me in the frame for the murder of both Morgane Avril and Myrtille Camus. I was the last one to have spoken to Piroz before he was knifed . . . And then there were all those grey areas in the Saint-Michel file.

After all, I was still the ideal scapegoat.

After all, perhaps I'd been lying since the start.

I held out my hand so that the young officer would lend me his shoulder. Where had those Fil Rouge idiots put my prosthesis? I suspected that over the next few hours I was going to have to relate, time and again, the unlikely sequence of events of the past six days.

And write it down as well, so as not to forget anything.

The worst along with the best.

The worst behind me, the best to come.

*

Remember. It was the first scene of this story.

I was having dinner with the prettiest girl in the world.

She had just put on a blue tulip dress. Her breasts danced naked and free beneath the silk of a low-cut top into which I could plunge my eyes for as long as I wanted.

Now I can tell you her name:

Océane.

I was about to make love with her.

Those were the first lines of this story, and they will be the last.

Thriller-lovers, sorry to disappoint you . . .

It's going to be a happy ending!

45

The best to come?

Champagne, Piper-Heidsieck, 2005 vintage.

Logs are on the fire, by a dark, low table of an exotic wood that I don't know, probably ridiculously expensive.

I'm sitting in a leather armchair of the same light-brown leather that they use to make Harley seats, gaucho boots, and the Stetsons that Texans wear. Worth a fortune! Being a gynaecologist must pay the bills.

Océane is making some noise in the kitchen. My coupe of Piper-Heidsieck is on the table, just beside the pile of a hundred sheets of paper – one hundred and thirteen, to be precise. The story of my last six days. I've printed it out for Océane to read, and when she's done, I'll close the file. For ever.

Who will open it again?

Who will read it?

Will it remain piece of introspection, forgotten at the back of a drawer? Will it become a breathtaking mystery novel with me as the main character?

Who will you be, you who are gazing at the text? Will you even exist?

Still uncertain of the answer, I decide to add a handwritten addendum to my diary, to bring it up to date.

The police freed Océane late in the afternoon. Her lawyer has said she won't face further charges. Self-defence. Confirmed by five witnesses. Frédéric Saint-Michel was going to shoot me, he would have killed me if Océane hadn't fired first. The police disciplinary body is still investigating Piroz's role in the affair. We'll all be called as witnesses, probably several times. Commander Weissman and three of his deputies, after hearing my story, looked at me with a kind of unhealthy pity and asked if I wanted to press charges.

Press charges? Against who?

They didn't seem to understand and let me go. The police have been quibbling, combing, scratching for two days, but I don't think they really care any more. They've got a culprit, a motive, some confessions, and more evidence than they need.

Frédéric Saint-Michel.

Arrested. Judged. Executed.

Case closed.

I arrived at Océane's place less than an hour ago. She lives in an isolated cottage in Lucy, a few kilometres from Neufchâtel-en-Bray, a doll's house with dovecotes and mud-brick walls, straw and irises on the roof, set between four hedges. A well, a pond, a labyrinth of gravel that runs between impeccably maintained flower beds. Carmen must spend hours in her daughter's garden.

Océane ushered me in, pointed me to the leather armchair and asked me to open the bottle of champagne while she went upstairs to change. When she came back down a few minutes later, she had swapped her pullover and jeans for a blue tulip dress.

The pen slipped from my hands. I felt the leather of the armchair melting beneath me.

A wide turquoise ribbon ran behind her neck before dividing into two strips of fabric that covered her breasts and then ran under her belt, with a breathtaking neckline. The flower-shaped dress escaped beneath the belt into a silk corolla that opened up on a pair of pretty pistils encased in lagoon-blue fishnet stockings.

She leaned over me, holding out a coupe, then disappeared to poke the fire. The dance of her long hair on her face seemed like a challenge to that of the flames in in the hearth.

I thought she was breathtakingly beautiful.

My heart was pounding fit to burst. To keep it from exploding, I focused my eyes on the curves of her dress. Océane was wearing nothing underneath, no parachute strap to help her escape, no bra.

She came towards me.

'Don't imagine that I'm just being nice to you so that you'll forgive me.'

Her lips pressed against mine as it to keep me from replying.

'You should have seen your face the day you came into my surgery in Neufchâtel. As if you'd seen a ghost.'

'An angel,' I murmured.

She held a finger vertically against my lips. Mockingly.

'And your adorable terror that morning when I jumped into the void from the cliff in Yport.'

'An angel,' I said again.

She clinked her champagne glass against mine.

'May I?'

Without asking my permission, she sat on my knees, delicately, with the flirtatious lightness of a little girl, as if to spare my artificial lightness. I held my breath.

'You're so . . .'

Again, she put her finger to my lips.

'Shhh . . .'

She stared at me with her coal-black eyes, at point-blank range. A showdown, eyelash to eyelash, until I gave in, until I lowered my eye to her breasts, barely concealed by the two turquoise curtains of sheer fabric. I resisted the desire to cover her breasts with my two hands, to follow the swell of them with my fingertips, to circle her dark areolas a thousand times. Still sitting on my knees, Océane swayed closer to me. Her breasts crushed against my torso as her crotch rubbed against the fly of my jeans.

I shivered.

The beautiful girl was wearing nothing under her dress.

Before I had time to wrap my arms around her waist, she sprang to her feet. Her fingers undid my belt and then, with the same movement, slipped my trousers and my boxer shorts down to my ankles.

I pleaded with God not to let the sight of my steel tibia put her off. She didn't even seem to notice. With the gesture of a princess she lifted her dress as if to avoid crumpling it when she sat down.

Her thighs parted gently.

Her lips trembled as I entered her body.

Océane's naked body was a cinema screen on which the wild shadows of the flames in the fireplace were projected.

'You haven't asked me the question,' I murmured in her ear.

The champagne ran down her throat. I felt a titillating desire to pour the bottle she was drinking from into the hollow of her neck, so that I could then plunge in my lips and tongue and drink.

'What question?'

'The one that everyone asks me. My leg. How did It happen? Before or after 2004?'

'I couldn't care less, Jamal.'

She pressed her hot body against me. I had never spoken seriously to an adult about my disability. And yet at that precise moment I no longer felt like playing, escaping, lying. After all, I would transcribe every word of this conversation with the woman of my dreams in the last lines of my story. My future readers also deserved to know the truth before the end.

I slid my hand along Océane's bare back and adopted a conspiratorial tone.

'Since I was born, I've spread dozens of versions, all different. I've even served up a few to the members of your Fil Rouge. Heroic exploits, tragic accidents. I was playing the crippled fireman, the unlucky robber, the reckless parkour athlete . . . But the truth is much simpler.'

Her hand rested tenderly on my shoulder as her lips kissed my neck.

'Some people are born with a twin sister – life multiplies everything by two.' I looked at her and smiled. 'For me, it divided everything in two. I was born with one kidney, one lung, one leg; one heart, of course, but it's too weak. My mother, Nadia, was forty-six when she fell pregnant, my father was over fifty. As far as they were concerned, I was their little miracle. During the first fifteen years of her married life, she had had a child every three years. Then nothing for the fifteen years that followed . . . Until I came along.'

Océane's kisses made their way down my chest, my caresses fell to the small of her back.

'My mother spent the last fifteen years of her life looking after me. By the time I was a teenager, I'd had eighteen operations. In total, I spent over twenty months in hospital. I put the social security budget 9.3 per cent deeper in deficit all on my own, at the age of ten. I grew up with the idea that I would never be an adult, that I hadn't enough parts in good condition in my engine to get very far along the road. That I was going to break down at any moment, and find myself abandoned by the side of the road. So I invented my future, I imagined the fate of an Achilles for myself – do you know what I mean? Accepting death, on condition that I would first enjoy life, fixing the bar not by numbering the years I had ahead of me, but the goals I had to achieve.'

'Do you have lots of those?' Océane murmured.

There was infinite tenderness in her voice. As if my confessions were arousing. I found myself regretting all the ridiculous versions I had been making up since my teenage years to seduce girls.

'Five . . . The five points of my star.'

She gently took the hand that I was running down her back and gripped it.

'As you can imagine, my mother wasn't about to let me go without a fight! A kidney, a lung, a decent heart – they exist, you can buy them, people donate them. She took her organ caddie around all the hospitals in France, she plagued the best surgeons. Operations costing millions of euros were billed to social security. Eighteen operations, just think. She gave me one of her lungs as soon as I had a thoracic cage the same size as hers, when I was fifteen. It was my last operation. The following winter finished off my mother.'

Her five fingers gripped mine.

'My last operation,' I said again. 'I was the man who cost three billion. Robocop, to my mates in La Courneuve. A completely new body, apart from a leg and a foot, the only part of the human body that no surgeon in the world had been able to graft on. But having only one foot doesn't keep you from moving forward as quickly as everyone else. Quicker, even. I started running on the day of my mother's funeral. I've never stopped.'

'I understand.'

'Everyone in the neighbourhood knows me. You just have to ask in any stairwell in La Courneuve. I've been ill from birth, I couldn't have been the rapist of Morgane and Myrtille.'

'Forgive us.'

I took advantage of the opportunity to steal a long kiss from her.

'You know, I've grown up one day at a time, with death on my heels. Every year in my letter to Santa, I would ask Father Christmas for one last year of life . . . So if you'd let me drown in Saint-Marcouf, basically I wouldn't have regretted a thing . . .'

'Not even the five directions of your star?'

I hesitated.

Had I changed? Had I given up on my ambitions?

I moved my hand from hers and rested it on her firm, round, full breast.

'My star can go on shining after my death, can't it?'

Océane shivered. Her hand took mine. She pressed it against her breast for a long time, then guided it over her skin, slowly, lower and lower to the edge of the world.

Océane slipped her dress back on over her head with a perfectly natural gesture. The silk enfolded her like a second skin.

'I'm hungry. Will you finish your journal while I put the final touches to our feast?'

Océane cooked?

I watched her crossing the room, mechanically picking up the champagne coupe to put it away, and then disappearing into the kitchen.

That was a few minutes ago.

361

Since then, sitting on the leather armchair, I'm faithfully transcribing every word, every gesture, every emotion that I felt during the hour that has just passed.

That's how my story will end.

In a few moments I will read it to Océane. We will probably make love again.

It's a lovely story, isn't it? The disabled Arab who everyone thought was guilty, finishing his life in the arms of the woman of his dreams. What do you think?

Probably too cute an ending for a thriller, I grant you. But what about a nice little romance? *Beauty and the Beast* . . .

I look up. Above a Norman dresser carved with fruit, a circular skylight with a lace curtain opens on to the sky. Stars sparkle against the pitch-dark background.

Which is mine?

Which will I use to find my bearings as I pursue the five points of my destiny?

My mind drifts to my previous life, the one I am about to rejoin on Monday, at the Saint Antoine Institute. Ibou, who will think I'm a lunatic, Ophélie, who will have collected new photographs of guys. That jerk Jérôme Pinelli, who will be green with envy.

Océane is singing in the kitchen. I think I recognise '*A nos actes manqués*' by Fredricks Goldman Jones. Can't swear to it.

My pen slows down on the white page. I have to be careful in choosing the last words in my story.

Have I won?

Has death finally stopped stalking me?

I hold my pen in the air for several seconds, until the sound of an oven door closing makes me turn my head. Océane appears holding a tea towel. A strong smell tickles my nose. Sauce chasseur, the one I wasn't allowed to try in the canteen. Mushrooms, shallots, cream and wine.

'Are you sure?' Océane says to me. 'You haven't told anyone where you are?'

'Absolutely certain!'

I've respected her privacy, I haven't told anyone about my visit to her house. This beautiful girl is probably ashamed of her awkward lover. Worried that Carmen won't approve. Afraid that Uncle Gilbert will complain. Afraid that Mona will make a scene?

Not Mona, Alina!

Jealous?

I love this air of mystery. The fact that our love is clandestine lends even more spice.

My pen rests on the page for the last time. I want to find a pretty phrase to end with. I'm slowing to a halt. I bite the cap of my biro.

'It's ready!' Océane calls.

Never mind. I'll go for the easy solution.

They were the first words of this story, and they will be the last.

For a long time, I was unlucky.

Fortune never favoured me.

To be completely honest, I still have trouble believing that it's swapped sides.

THE END

IV
Execution

From: Gérard Calmette, Director of the Disaster Victim Identification Unit (DVIU), Criminal Research Institute of the National Gendarmerie, Rosny-sous-Bois

To: Lieutenant Bertrand Donnadieu, National Gendarmerie, Territorial Brigade of the District of Étretat, Seine-Maritime

Dear Lieutenant,

I am sending you this brief letter to inform you about one particular issue raised by the case of the three skeletons found on 12 July 2014 on the beach at Yport. I may succinctly remind you that these three individuals, whom we have named, for the purposes of the inquiry, Albert, Bernard and Clovis, died at different dates: Albert during the summer of 2004; Bernard between autumn 2004 and winter 2005; Clovis between February and March 2014, and that the cause of their deaths is criminal poisoning with muscarine, a dose which according to experts led to the death of each of the three individuals, through cardiac arrest, less than thirty minutes after the absorption of the poison.

But as research progresses, we find ourselves confronted with a strange detail that obliges me to ask you a question for which I apologise in advance, Lieutenant.

Might your forces have neglected to send us one of the pieces of evidence from this inquiry? To put it another way, we are missing one of

the pieces of the puzzle and ask you to check very carefully that it has not gone missing.

Let me explain. We have been able to reconstruct the skeletons of Albert and Bernard in their entirety from the bones that you have given us. This is a precise piece of palaeontological work, but one to which we are accustomed.

On the other hand, in spite of our efforts, we have not succeeded in completely reconstructing the skeleton of Clovis which, may I remind you, is the name given to the individual who died most recently, in February 2014, a few days after the Avril–Camus case was solved by the death of the alleged double murderer, Frédéric Saint-Michel. I use the adjective 'alleged' because, in my previous letter, I categorically indicated that the DNA of Albert, poisoned in the summer of 2004, corresponded to that of the sperm found on the bodies and clothes of Morgane Avril and Myrtille Camus. As things stand, I have had no reply from Judge Lagarde, to whom I sent a copy of my previous letter.

Clovis's skeleton corresponds to that of a man less than thirty years old, perfectly proportioned, who had died six months previously, in a very advanced state of decomposition. When we attempted to assemble the bones that you sent us, in spite of our most advanced research, combinations and investigations, we were obliged to admit the obvious.

The skeleton lacks a tibia.

In the hope that you may be able to supply an explanation for this missing or lost part, please accept my cordial regards,

Gérard Calmette
Director, DVIU

46

Have I won?

Océane closed the boot of the Audi Q3 without a glance at Jamal's body. She merely checked that no one could be watching them in the darkness of the garden. The only light came from a lamp post at the end of the street whose halo was not bright enough to pierce the hedges surrounding the courtyard.

It was cold. Fine snow fell in a damp layer on the roofs and pavements. Nobody would be going out this evening. Océane would have free rein to transport the body to join the others.

She went back to the shelter of her cottage.

Of the three, Jamal was the one she had been most reluctant to kill. She didn't even include Piroz in her tally; he didn't count. She had been forced to eliminate him because he had worked it all out. Drunk as he was, it had taken her less than a minute to stick a knife in him and tip him over the railing of the *Paramé*.

She walked towards the fireplace. A few flames lingered on the burnt-out logs.

Jamal Salaoui was a different matter. Objectively, he didn't deserve to die. He was a victim, like her. A victim of the system, of the judgement of others and their copy-cat violence. A scapegoat in the most accurate sense of the word, an innocent who assumes the collective guilt of everyone else.

Of all other men.

Océane walked over to the low table and picked up Jamal's story, more than a hundred pages, and threw it in the fire. Nothing

369

happened at first, and then the paper ignited like a huge torch.

Jamal Salaoui would have kept thinking it over until he discovered the truth.

Thanks to Piroz, he'd learned how to solve the prisoner's dilemma – it was all there in Jamal's diary. Even if Jamal himself hadn't worked it out, an astute reader could have put a different construction on the clues he had missed, and wondered about the inconsistences in the official version. Understood.

Océane dropped her tulip dress. For several seconds she stood naked by the fireplace, letting the heat of the flames devour her skin. She savoured that moment when no man could rest his eyes on her body, or desire her like an object to be possessed.

Never again will a boy come between us.

Morgane's voice echoed faintly in her head. Her sister was seven years old, they had both been climbing in the big apple tree outside their mother's holiday cottage. It was springtime, and blossom fell into their hair and on to their shoulders, a fairy-tale pink rain.

Never again will a boy come between us.

They had promised. They wouldn't need a knight, a prince or a king to become princesses. They were sisters, twins, one for all and all for one. Nothing could ever slip between them.

Not so much as a petal.

The fire was already dying in the hearth. Only a few scraps of Jamal's diary were still floating around. Océane bent down and picked up the ashes to rekindle the flickering flames. She had to be careful, as she had been for the last ten years. Of course, nice obedient Jamal hadn't told anyone he was coming to see her, but when the police discovered that he was missing, they were bound to question her. She could leave no sign that he had been there. Still less of his diary.

The twins had carried on climbing the apple tree until they turned eighteen. They had promised, every spring, every year, and it had brought them closer and made them stronger, more beautiful too.

No boy between them. Ever.

In turn they were Snow White and her mirror. Siamese princesses. Two hearts, one blood.

Their mother, with only one heart, had never needed a man. She had made a family, all by herself. She had built with her own hands the most beautiful house in Neufchâtel-en-Bray, all by herself. She had taken power at the council, at the Pays de Bray development association, all by herself. No man had ever come between the mother and her daughters.

The fire had gone out. Océane let the cold make the hairs on her skin stand up, then climbed to her room to put on a pair of black jeans and a dark pullover. It was time for Jamal Salaoui's body to join the other two.

The roads of the Pays de Caux were deserted. The cold rain whitened the slopes and the skeletons of the trees. Océane ran no risk of being stopped by the police. Who could venture out at three o'clock in the morning, on secondary roads swept by the wind and the icy drizzle? In the light of the headlights, a sign pointed towards Yport. Ten kilometres.

Morgane's promise echoed around her head again.

Never again will a boy come between us.

The riffs of the guitars at the party on 5 June 2004 crashed in her brain. Images ran through her mind, against a background of deafening music. The trip to Yport with Clara, Nicolas, Mathieu and Morgane. The night at the Sea View. The dance floor.

The windscreen wipers beat along with the rhythm of her heart, crushing her tears, which still came back, each time heavier than before.

No boy between us. Ever.

Océane had repeated it to her. She had murmured it in her ear, in Nicolas's Clio, when she had noticed Morgane changing in the back seat and putting on that dress that clung to her breasts and bottom. She had yelled it at her on the dance floor, parting the forest of wolf-eyed men encircling her sister. The techno music thumped. Morgane, in a trance, hadn't heard. Hadn't listened. Hadn't even looked.

But Morgane had promised . . .

Nicolas and Clara were kissing on the sofa. That idiot Mathieu had even tried his luck, had put a hand on her thigh, brushed his lips against her neck. Did he think she was going to renege on her promise, for a cockroach like him? He had fallen asleep over his vodka and orange. Océane had been drinking as well. A lot. Much too much. More than she had ever drunk in her life.

Then she had followed them.

Morgane had chosen one of the wolves. Not a leader of the pack, more of a cub with milk teeth, his shirt open over a hairless chest, and with a ridiculous red scarf around his neck.

Océane had seen them kissing in the car park, undressing at the end of the beach. In the shadow of the cliff, she had heard them running towards the sea, stifling their laughter, touching each other in the water, coming back out shivering. Hiding behind the sea wall, she had heard Morgane sighing under the stranger's caresses, holding back her moans, giving herself, forgetting herself.

You promised, a voice screamed in her head, *no boy, ever.* Then they had got dressed – Morgane hadn't even taken the time to put her panties back on. Océane, tottering, had followed her sister and the boy with the scarf to the blockhouse. Which of the two had taken the other's hand to lead them up there, to gaze out at the sea and the cliff? Océane had never known.

When she'd looked out at the view, the slate roofs of the houses of Yport had taunted her like grey waves. A few minutes later, when the wolf cub had departed, Océane had emerged from her hiding place. Morgane was wearing the stranger's scarf around her neck.

'Alex gave it to me.'

His name was Alexandre. Alexandre Da Costa.

'It's our connection. Our red thread. We're going to see each other again. He's not like the oth—'

*

372

Her tears were unstoppable now. Océane slowed down, then parked on the edge of the road, just before the Bénouville junction. The images were too powerful. Blurred. They jostled one another.

Her cries in the night. Morgane's smile.

You didn't have the right. You promised me.

Morgane's laughter.

No boy. No boy between us. Ever.

Her defiant laughter.

Océane saw her fingers tearing Morgane's dress, her hands tightening the scarf to make her stop laughing, to make her weep, to make her plead for forgiveness and then snuggle in her arms, to promise . . .

No man would ever come between them again.

Océane saw Morgane's eyes freeze, her body tumbling down the slope, tipping over the edge and into the void.

The Audi set off again, slowly. Thousands of times Océane had replayed the moment when Morgane's eyes had looked into hers, the life in them ebbing away, before she had flown away from her into the void. Which of them, the princess or her mirror, had died that evening?

Neither? Both?

The police hadn't been able to make sense of it. On the beach they had discovered a pretty girl, strangled, her dress torn, traces of sperm on her body and in her vagina, the signs of recent penetration and violent assault. What other conclusion could their pathetic minds arrive at? It had to be rape! Océane felt nothing but contempt for their incompetence.

The Audi passed Bénouville. The village was asleep. Perhaps it slept all winter long. A sign warned drivers: 'Valleuse du Curé – No entry.' Océane turned the car and drove another hundred metres or so along a dirt road. Who would think of coming here to look for Jamal Salaoui's body? Nobody, any more than they'd thought of coming here for the other two, ten years ago. By tomorrow morning the rain would have erased all trace of tyres on the path.

*

Océane had had no trouble finding Alexandre Da Costa. He was hiding in Blonville-sur-Mer in the second home of his parents, a couple who'd taken early retirement so they could spend nine months of the year in the Caribbean, in Saint-Vincent-et-les-Grenadines. He might have been stupid, but even he understood that he was the prime suspect in the rape and murder of Morgane Avril, thanks to his DNA and his Burberry scarf.

He knew he risked arrest if he ventured out of his hiding place, but Océane had lured him out with a phone call, claiming she'd had a text from her sister right before she was murdered, naming Alexandre Da Costa as her lover.

The moron told Océane that some man must have attacked Morgane as soon as he left her, perhaps to steal her handbag. She assured him that she hadn't reported him to the police, she wanted to talk to him first. She wanted to understand. She wanted to know all of her sister's emotions that night. They agreed to meet at a roadside motel in Yvetot, where you check in via a machine and never have to deal with a human being. He came running, like a good little doggie. Tail between his legs at first, then a bit more cocky.

He was startled by her beauty, the idiot. He found her even more beautiful than her sister, the monster. Less demonstrative, perhaps, on the mattress in room 301, but then his heart stopped beating under the effects of the muscarine added to that horrible moussaka reheated in the microwave in the hall. Océane had carefully slipped between her fingers the condom containing his sperm and emptied it into a glass bottle. Then at 3 a.m. she loaded the body into the boot of her car and drove away.

'No man will ever come between us,' she had murmured to the stars, letting his corpse drop into the darkness.

It was three long months before Alexandre Da Costa's parents reported the disappearance of their twenty-two-year-old son. They only heard from him once or twice a year, they had no idea where he lived; in addition to their house in Normandy, they had two other residences in France, one on the Côte d'Azur and the other on the Île de Ré, a third on the island of Cres in Croatia and a flat in the Balearics. Océane had since learned that sixty-five thousand people disappeared in France every year, and that more than ten thousand of those were never found . . .

No one would ever make the connection.

Carmen Avril would spend the rest of her life looking for her daughter's murderer, seeking vengeance. All for nothing. He was dead. Océane had already avenged her sister. The man who had tried to separate them, both of them, all three, slept for all eternity in a hole in the depths of the cliff.

Océane parked the Audi Q3 behind a clump of ash trees, taking care that no late-night hiker wandering in the fields – in the unlikely event of such a person existing – would spot her car. Now came the hardest part.

She loaded the body on to her shoulders, taking care to leave no trace, no fingerprint, no hair, no drop of sweat. Then she set off to walk the last hundred and fifty metres.

Ten years earlier, in June 2004, before arranging to meet Alexandre Da Costa, Océane had spent days wandering the cliffs. Passers-by and police officers who passed her assumed she was collecting her thoughts. Some may have imagined she was thinking of jumping off the cliff to join her twin. How could they have guessed that she was looking for a pit that would swallow up inconvenient men and make them disappear? A pit big enough to throw half of humanity into.

She had found it a little way east of Bénouville, near the Fond d'Étigues: a sinkhole hidden between the brambles, known only to the cows.

Océane held her breath as she opened the boot. She had rolled Jamal's body up in a blanket that she would burn as soon as she got back to Neufchâtel.

It was the third time in her life that she had parked her car here.

The incredible news had come on 27 August 2004. A girl had been found raped, strangled with a red Burberry scarf, in Lower Normandy. One Myrtille Camus. General panic. The serial killer had struck a second time. And he would do it again . . .

Océane's mother had called a meeting of the Fil Rouge that very evening, in the canteen at the school in Grandcamp-Maisy that the mayor had cleared for the occasion. She wanted to meet all the relatives of this girl Myrtille, her best friend, her future husband. Time was pressing. They would have to catch the killer before he could escape. Or start again. Collect as many clues as possible. The police had already shown that they couldn't be trusted to find the killer; if they had, Myrtille would still be alive.

Counting Uncle Gilbert, there were eight people around the table. Three on the Avril side, five on the Camus side.

During the journey from Neufchâtel to Grandcamp, while Uncle Gilbert drove, cursing Parisian drivers under his breath, and her mother ranted about catching the bastard who'd killed her daughter, Océane had come to the conclusion that Myrtille Camus had been murderered by someone close to her. Why else would he have disguised his crime and directed suspicion at the notorious 'red-scarf killer'?

Only two people knew that there was no serial killer: Océane, and the murderer of Myrtille Camus.

When Uncle Gilbert parked his old Mercedes E-Class in the school car park at Grandcamp-Maisy for that first meeting of the Fil Rouge, Océane had struggled to hide her excitement. Among the five people sitting with them around the table, was one the murderer of Myrtille Camus?

Océane dropped Jamal's body. Her back was on fire. She hadn't gone thirty metres and already she was exhausted. She'd never manage to carry him to the pit. She took time to think. She'd have to drag him the rest of the way. Drag him and then clear up after herself. She took a deep breath.

Her mind returned again to Grandcamp-Maisy and that meeting with the Camus family. That evening she had made a mistake, the only one in ten years. A mistake that would cost her dear.

As soon as she had stepped into the school canteen and stared at the five people sitting behind the octagonal table, Océane had suspected Frédéric Saint-Michel of having killed his fiancée. None of the other people close to her looked like a credible culprit. She had studied Chichin all evening, keeping an eye on his smallest gestures, each quiver, as he listened to Carmen summarising the police reports.

Before the hour was up, she knew it was him.

But she had forgotten one important detail.

Myrtille Camus's murderer had exactly the same advantage. He too knew that the serial killer was a chimera. He was therefore alert to the possibility he could be in the presence of Morgane's murderer.

When their eyes met, without even saying a word to each other, they had understood. Océane had given herself away by studying him too intently. Who could have suspected him? Who could have doubted the theory of the serial killer other than someone who knew that Morgane hadn't been killed an unknown opportunist, striking at random?

Who but her murderer?

They were bound by a pact of silence.

While assessing the best way of gripping Jamal's corpse, Océane thought again of that theorem dug up by Piroz – the prisoner's dilemma. Two accomplices, who can give each other way, or not. If they denounce one another, they lose everything. If they say nothing and cooperate, they both win. Until one of the two is sure that he can betray without the other one having the chance to retaliate. Maximum gain, according to the theory. Piroz was anything but stupid, as policemen went. He had guessed right, but his voice carried a little too far when he'd been drinking, and she'd heard every word through the thin partition walls of the *Paramé*.

On the evening of the murder of Myrtille Camus, the first meeting of the Fil Rouge had finished at midnight. Just before heading back to the car, where Uncle Gilbert was waiting to drive them back to the hotel, Océane had gone to use the toilet down the corridor from the canteen. Frédéric Saint-Michel had joined her there. White as a sheet.

'It was an accident,' he had stammered in a low voice. 'An accident. I didn't mean to strangle her. We were supposed to get married. She loved me, she would never have left me. That guy didn't matter to her. Myrtille loved me. We made love one last time just before—'

'With a condom, I hope?'

Saint-Michel had stared at her. He was no better than any other man. At that moment Océane was already thinking about eliminating him, like Da Costa. She would do it as soon as she could, but it was too risky to act now.

'Yes,' he had admitted.

'I've got a present for you!'

Océane had taken the glass bottle out of her pocket. Saint-Michel, of course, hadn't understood.

'The man who raped my sister gave it to me,' Océane explained. 'But you're going to have to tell me more before I let you have it.'

Saint-Michel's hands had closed on the bottle while he murmured words of confession as if speaking to a priest. Panicking after his fiancée's murder, he had hidden Myrtille's body under the ferns in the Grandes Carrières, hoping that no one would find it before he came back. Then, knowing that he would be suspected as soon as his fiancée's body had been identified, he had come up with the idea of copying the Yport murder which had been dominating every front page the last couple of months. Saint-Michel had driven to Deauville, gone into the Burberry shop in the shopping centre, bought a €150 shirt to allay the suspicions of the salesgirls while he slipped a red cashmere scarf into his pocket. On a deserted beach on the way back, he had filled a jerry-can with seawater to splash over Myrtille's body. Finally, once he was back in Grandes Carrières, he had taken her handbag and her panties, precisely reproducing the actions of the murderer of Morgane Avril. Only one detail was missing, the Moleskine notebook in which Myrtille recorded her intimate thoughts. He could find no trace of it, either on her or in her handbag.

Their conversation had been interrupted by Carmen Avril's voice ringing out from the other end of the corridor.

'Shall we go, Océane?'

'I'm coming, Mum.'

Océane had let Saint-Michel keep the glass bottle.

Cooperation–reciprocity.

That simple offering cleared them both.

The next morning, the police found Myrtille Camus's panties hooked among the brambles a few hundred metres from Grandes Carrières, stained with the rapist's sperm, identical to the sperm found in Morgane Avril's vagina.

The ultimate proof that there was only one killer.

A serial killer who chose his victims at random.

Océane puffed again. She had dragged Jamal's body about a hundred metres. Just another twenty to go and it would all be over. Only a few stars and a quarter-moon lit the fields as far as the eye could see. The drizzle had intensified. It would erase any tracks. In the morning there wouldn't be a trace. Océane turned up the hood of her coat, rubbed her gloved hands and went back to work.

On 6 October 2004, late in the afternoon, Océane had the good fortune to be manning the Fil Rouge phone line. Knowing that many potential witnesses would be hesitant about talking to the police, the association had advertised a number where anyone with information could speak in the strictest confidence.

Olivier Roy had a shy voice.

'I'm the one everyone's looking for,' he had snivelled. 'The boy with the Adidas cap, the one who was prowling around Myrtille. The one the police—'

Océane had told him to be quiet, not to tell a soul. She had wanted to meet up with him at the roadside motel in Yvetot that evening, but he had refused. Too far, too late, too dangerous. Instead she had arranged to meet him the following morning in the Veys Marshlands a few kilometres from his house, in an abandoned hunting lodge.

'I didn't kill her, madame,' he had wailed down the phone. 'Everyone thinks I did, but I didn't kill her. I loved her. She was going to leave her guy. She wrote me poems. She wrote them in her diary.'

'Have you got that diary?'

'Yes, but . . .'

'Bring it.'

Olivier Roy, like everyone else, thought Myrtille Camus had been the victim of a vagrant. He had no reason to suspect his rival, Chichin. He had been trying to get up the courage to hand himself in to the police. He had spent his days worrying about what to do and thinking about Myrtille. He would never have hurt her, he was completely innocent. But the police had posted up a photofit that vaguely looked like him, and he was afraid they would ignore his pleas of innocence and find him guilty. He had decided to contact the Fil Rouge because he'd heard they had lawyers and investigators working for them; he believed they would listen to him, they would advise him, tell him how to deal with the cops.

In the hunting lodge, Oliver had given Océane all the souvenirs that he had kept of Myrtille: her Moleskine notebook, her letters, her poems. He was so relieved to hand them over, as if a burden had been lifted. Not half as relieved as Océane. If Olivier Roy had talked, suspicions would have fallen on Frédéric Saint-Michel. If Frédéric Saint-Michel fell, she would fall with him . . .

Never again will a boy come between us.

Océane had opened her bag. It was midday and the sun was reaching its zenith above the marsh. Ducks and woodcocks nested in the rust-coloured bog. Olivier seemed to think it was beautiful. He struck Océane as romantic, depressive, completely out of his depth. When she took out a bottle of Coke, some slices of cold pizza and oriental pastries, he had been delighted to share her picnic. He must have found everything curiously spicy. Not for long. His eyes had grown heavy, his breathing had slowed, then, like a hunting dog waiting for its master's whistle, he had frozen. His heart had stopped beating.

The next day, Saint-Michel had received a poem written by his late fiancée. Océane was playing the game.

Cooperation—reciprocity.

Saint-Michel was clever; he had shared the contents of the letter with Commander Bastinet. A preventive measure.

Meanwhile, little Alina, thinking about the last days of her best friend, was asking more and more questions.

Another twenty metres. Océane walked forward cautiously, careful to part the brambles without getting stuck on them. The police might be stupid, but they were persistent. A scrap of fabric caught on a thorn could lead them to identify whoever it was who had come here to dispose of their rubbish.

With the disappearance of Olivier Roy, the investigation had deflated like a balloon. In spite of Carmen's fury, the police had dropped the case. They had passed it to the gendarmerie in Fécamp, and in particular to Captain Piroz, who was keeping the flame alive.

Back to square one.

Carmen had become obsessed with the search for the stranger who was in Yport and in Isigny on the dates of the murders . . . Océane did nothing to stop her. After all, it was the only thing stopping her mother from going completely mad.

Meanwhile Océane had taken the precaution of approaching Alina Masson, Myrtille Camus's best friend, and sowing doubt in her mind. Just enough to prepare her for the day when they would have to get rid of Saint-Michel. It was as if she were introducing malware, a Trojan horse on the brain's hard drive, with each insidious question.

What if Myrtille hadn't been killed by a vagrant?
What if Myrtille knew her killer?

Then, in March 2013, a name had finally emerged from the big tombola: Jamal Salaoui. At last they'd found their man. Only Océane and Saint-Michel knew that the poor wretch who'd had the misfortune to be in both wrong places at the wrong time was innocent.

When Carmen had drawn up her crazy plan to unmask Salaoui, Océane had gone along with it. This was the opportunity she had been waiting for to break with Saint-Michel. The grand finale in Saint-Marcouf had been her suggestion. She had gone there ahead of time to dislodge a brick from the wall of the citadel and hide Myrtille Camus's notebook in it. Then she'd carved M2O on the brick and replaced it. Using Alina as her courier, she'd supplied Jamal Salaoui with a series of brown envelopes filled with clues so that he would understand, just when they needed him to . . . Then she paid a visit to Frédéric Saint-Michel's apartment, using a key she'd stolen from him years previously during one of the endless Fil Rouge meetings, to hide Morgane's handbag in a drawer, and to plant a glass bottle containing traces of Alexandre Da Costa's sperm – a smaller sample than the one she'd given to Saint-Michel in 2004, but enough for the police laboratory to run their tests.

Early the next day she threw herself off the cliff in front of Jamal Salaoui, for a 120-metre drop slowed only by a pocket parachute. Jamal Saloui's fate had been decided, and no one, not even Piroz, could save him.

That economist, Axelrod, had been wrong about his pseudo-method for solving the prisoner's dilemma.

Cooperation–reciprocity–pardon.

It only worked if the accomplices met up again once they were out of prison, and wanted to collaborate again. Or take their revenge. The correct method was to betray only once, once and for all.

Blow for blow. Shoot first.

Cooperation–betrayal–punishment.

Océane went on dragging Jamal's body closer to the hole. By her calculation, it was about thirty metres deep, perhaps more if one took into account the tunnels that snaked beneath the chalk. Doubtless some local farmers knew the site, perhaps even made use of it to get rid of inconvenient objects. But it wouldn't have occurred to them to climb down into the pit.

Perhaps some caver would go down there in fifty years from now and find the three skeletons in among the carcases of dogs, old television sets and rusty washing machines. Or in a hundred years, when the cliff had retreated enough. It didn't matter when the bodies were found – even if they were found tomorrow – no one would ever be able to establish a connection between those three corpses and Océane. Even if they succeeded in identifying the remains, reconstructing the date of their death and the manner of their murder – modern forensic methods would allow them to do that much – there was nothing to connect them to her.

They had all fallen into the spider's web – she hadn't even had to draw them into it.

She repeated one last time, like a prayer: 'Never again will a boy come between us.' Now it was a certainty. All the men had paid. All the men who had approached her, who had approached them both, were dead.

She untied the cords and unrolled the blanket. Jamal's corpse rolled gently over the purple fabric, as if on a carpet that had been unrolled in front of him for one last ceremony. His body slipped silently into the bottomless hole.

It was over.

Océane was in a hurry to get back to Neufchâtel-en-Bray, but she had to take care, check that she hadn't left any trace of her presence in the faint light of the torch that barely lit the tips of her feet.

Couldn't wait to get home.

Couldn't wait to see her mother again.

Océane looked through the pale halo at the bare and stunted silhouettes of the chestnut trees lashed by the sea wind.

Couldn't wait for the apple tree by the Dos-d'Âne to blossom again.

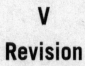

V
Revision

Fécamp, 13 August 2014

From: Lieutenant Bertrand Donnadieu, National Gendarmerie, Territorial Brigade of the District of Étretat, Seine-Maritime

To: Gérard Calmette, Director of the Disaster Victim Identification Unit (DVIU), Criminal Research Institute of the National Gendarmerie, Rosny-sous-Bois

Dear Monsieur Calmette,
In reply to your letter of 10 August 2014 concerning the identification of the three skeletons, Albert, Bernard and Clovis, found on the beach at Yport on 12 July 2014, and your concern regarding 'a missing piece of the puzzle', I would like to reassure you. The tibia of the skeleton named as Clovis has not been lost, either by your forces or by mine, nor carried away by the sea after the collapse of the cliff.
Reading your letter, we could not help making the connection with one of the chief protagonists in the Avril–Camus case, Jamal Salaoui, a young man who was for some time suspected of being the rapist and murderer of the two girls. You will easily understand the reasons for our deduction. Jamal Salaoui suffered from a disability, and a prosthesis replaced the lower part of his left leg. But more importantly, this young man disappeared six months ago, some days after the resolution of the Avril–Camus case. For no apparent reason. With no explanation.
Undeniably, your discovery reopens the case. Clearly, for reasons unknown, Jamal Salaoui was murdered.

To be frank, we were not entirely confident about the outcome of this investigation, even though it called into question the conclusions of the Avril–Camus case. It would be difficult to accuse the double rapist Frédéric Saint-Michel of this poisoning, in view of the fact that he was shot on the Île Saint-Marcouf three days before the disappearance of Jamal Salaoui! No other actor in this tragedy has aroused our suspicions. Whoever he may be, the individual who poisoned these three men acted in a particularly meticulous, methodical and prudent manner.

In response to your letter, we relaunched our investigation into the disappearance of Jamal Salaoui, jointly conducted at the time with the gendarmerie in Fécamp and the regional crime squad in Rouen. We questioned everyone close to Salaoui: relatives, cousins and friends, as well as the other protagonists in the Avril–Camus case, the members of the now defunct Fil Rouge Association, and finally his colleagues at the Saint Antoine Therapeutic Institute. No one knew anything. Jamal Salaoui was a secretive and introverted young man who had constructed an imaginary world around himself, a kind of bubble to which very few people were admitted. His superior, Jérôme Pinelli, described him as a potential depressive. But even he had to admit it was out of the question that Salaoui could have poisoned himself with muscarine and then thrown himself into a hole in the cliff to join two other bodies that had died by the same method years earlier.

We were about to get into our cars to leave the Saint Antoine Institute when one last witness came forward. A fifteen-year-old female inmate called to us from her third-floor window. The staff had isolated her in her room for the duration of our visit, but she was determined to speak to us.

Staff warned us that the girl, Ophélie Parodi, was psychologically unstable and suffered from serious sexual disturbances linked to her childhood. She had developed a crush on Jamal Salaoui, who had been warned several times to keep his distance from her. Her behaviour – screaming and lashing out hysterically at the staff members trying to restrain her – certainly seemed unstable, but I insisted on hearing what she had to say.

As it turned out, little Ophélie had nothing to tell us . . . but she did have something to show us: her mobile phone.

She had received a text. The sender's first name, Jamal, was framed by two smiley emojis.

It was sent on 25 February 2014. 9.18 p.m. The day of Salaoui's disappearance. No one had seen him since – or not until six months later, when his decomposed corpse was recovered. So this young inmate was the last person to have been in contact with Salaoui.

The text itself was, to say the least, cryptic.

20 out of 20?

It was accompanied by a picture. A candid snapshot showing a woman in a blue tulip dress, a tea towel in her hand, in a kitchen.

Though the photograph was somewhat blurred and taken from behind the subject, showing her face in quarter-profile, there is no question as to her identity.

Océane Avril. The sister of the first victim.

I had questioned her several times about the disappearance of Salaoui. She struck me as an intelligent woman who showed real dignity in spite of the ordeal that she had been through. I saw no reason whatsoever to suspect her of any wrongdoing.

I immediately ordered that she be placed under arrest. Océane Avril is currently being held at the Vignettes detention centre in Val-de-Reuil. The preliminary psychiatric reports are damning.

Since then, forensic computer experts have managed to recover a number of deleted files from Jamal Salaoui's laptop. Among them, an account written in the days that followed the supposed resolution of the Avril–Camus case. I have read it, and it is very edifying. Intercut this manuscript with our correspondence, Monsieur Calmette, and you will have a story that any publisher would be in a great hurry to publish. Little Salaoui deserved as much, in the end.

I cannot resist giving you one last piece of evidence, Monsieur Calmette, even though it adds nothing more to the case. Young Ophélie Parodi had replied almost immediately to the text sent by Jamal Salaoui. According to our reconstruction of events, Salaoui had already ingested the muscarine by this time, and his death was inevitable.

The message was brief. It echoed a message sent by Jamal Salaoui to

Ophélie some days previously. Whatever the psychiatrists at the Saint Antoine Institute might say, this girl, although emotionally disturbed, is far from stupid. Her response to the photograph of Océane Avril and the question Salaoui had posed, '20 out of 20?' was two lines long:

Too beautiful. Beware of appearances.
I preferred the redhead.

Now you know everything.
  With cordial regards,
  Bertrand Donnadieu,
  Territorial Brigade of the District of Étretat

Eighteen days later, 31 August 2014

Émile opened cabin 22 of the cable car of the Aiguille du Midi to release the sixty Chinese tourists, their legs still wobbly after a journey spent hanging from a wire above a two-thousand-metre drop.

He took three steps towards the edge and lit a Marlboro.

Eight p.m. Any other day, this would have been his final task. He'd be locking up and heading off for a well-earned beer on the terrace of the Choucas.

Not today.

The little redhead let the last of the Chinese visitors pass and then walked towards him. Behind her stood a well-built man, handsome as a mountain infantryman, less tanned, but wearing the same snow-white coat with badges and braids. Very classy. Probably someone from the Office of Public Prosecutions, Émile thought.

He extended a hand to the girl. 'Mademoiselle Alina Masson?'

The girl slipped her hand into his.

'No. Salinas. Mona Salinas.'

Émile shrugged. If the minister had made a mistake, he didn't care. The bodyguard of the OPP gave him a series of authorisations with red, white and blue stamps. Émile spat out the stub of his cigarette, and then pointed to the sliding door of the cable car.

'It's leaving. Last one of the day . . . I'll get in with you. What you are asking me to do, mademoiselle, is something unprecedented, as far as I know.'

The cable car shook. The two black cables looked like two enormous scratches that disfigured the mountain all the way to its snowy peaks, almost three thousand metres higher. Mona was holding her treasure to her chest. Hervé, the representative of the Directory of Criminal Matters and Pardons, was made of marble.

'This is crazy, this business,' Émile went on, if only to fill the silence. 'It may even be forbidden.'

Hervé chimed in: 'Authorisation is granted directly by the minister. You are aware of the story, aren't you? Don't you think it's touching?'

Émile stared at Mont Blanc without replying.

Touching.

If the muscle-men of the ministry are getting their tissues out . . .

'Given the circumstances,' Hervé went on, 'the ministry would find it difficult to refuse this symbolic gesture by Mademoiselle Masson.'

'I thought her name was Salinas,' the cable car conductor muttered into his beard.

Due north, the last rays of the sun painted the Vallée Blanche with pink and gold reflections. Émile turned on his walkie-talkie.

'Next stop requested! Étoile station. Paradise Road exit right under our feet.'

A moment later the cabin came to a standstill. Mona smiled, staring at the sky. Émile crouched down on the floor and unscrewed a security trapdoor.

Thirty centimetres by thirty.

Four bolts.

A void of more than one thousand one hundred metres below their feet.

Mona took her eyes off the sky and lowered her gaze to the Vallée de Chamonix.

'Where are the racers going past?' she asked.

'Down there,' Hervé replied gently. 'Behind the Aiguille de Bionnassay, that white pyramid along the crest. They will pass through the Col du Tricot a little lower down. I've run the north face twice, that's probably why they've entrusted me with this mission. The runners set off just over two hours ago. The first should reach Italy before nightfall. Then they will have another fifteen hours of running, the fastest of them.'

Émile sighed, as if the effort of the participants in the Mont Blanc Ultra-Trail was nothing in comparison with the effort he was making to deal with the four bolts that couldn't have been unscrewed for an eternity.

Mona slowly turned the lid of the urn.

Just above her, Venus was already shining. Five dreams . . . She spread the fingers of her left hand and recited them one by one, murmuring them silently like one last prayer.

Five dreams. Jamal would have accomplished them all.

To be mourned by a woman when I die, Mona whispered.

Tears ran down her cheeks. She bent her thumb. Hervé offered her a handkerchief, which she refused.

To pay my debt before I die.

Bending her index finger, Mona thought of the arrest of Océane Avril, accused of six murders: the three bodies found in the cliff, that bastard Saint-Michel, Captain Piroz, Morgane, her twin . . . Jamal had managed to reveal the truth, the truth that had defeated a thousand police officers over ten years. She closed her eyes, and her memories drifted towards a swing in an empty playground above the beach at Yport. The first time she had heard of Ophélie. They had talked a lot about Jamal since then. Next weekend, the Saint Antoine Institute had agreed to let the girl spend two days with her, in Elbeuf.

Three bolts rolled on the floor of the cable car. Émile was triumphant. The wind blew behind the metal plaque.

'As soon as I've released the last one, it's going to shake.'

Mona shivered in spite of herself.

*

Make love to a woman more beautiful than me.

She closed her middle finger. The images of that first night in the Sirène passed in front of her. Room 7. The sound of pebbles rolled by the waves. Their skin. Her recklessness. Making love without a condom.

An icy blast abruptly engulfed the cabin. Émile held the iron plate in his hands.

'Alina,' Hervé said. 'Let's get this over with.'

His voice was less gentle, more pressing.

Mona closed her ring finger.

Have a child.

For a moment her hand touched her round belly as the high-altitude currents rocked the cabin. Six months since that night in the Sirène.

She gently knelt down by the trapdoor. Hervé held her back by the shoulder but there was no danger. No body, however slender, could have passed through that opening. She tipped the urn towards the void below.

Become the first disabled athlete to run the Mont Blanc Ultra-Trail.

She bent her little finger and, with her right hand, poured the ashes through the trapdoor.

The wind immediately scattered them towards the Blanc du Tacul, the Mont Maudit and the Dômes de Miage, high, very high, at a rate and an altitude that would never reach the runners of the Ultra-Trail whose multicoloured ski suits could been seen on the path that ran along the Glacier des Bossons.